Prosthetic Joi

Trisha Peel
Editor

Prosthetic Joint Infections

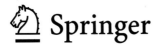 Springer

Editor
Trisha Peel
Department of Infectious Diseases
Monash University and Alfred Health
Melbourne, Victoria
Australia

ISBN 978-3-319-65249-8   ISBN 978-3-319-65250-4   (eBook)
https://doi.org/10.1007/978-3-319-65250-4

Library of Congress Control Number: 2017960822

This Springer imprint is published by Springer Nature
The registered company is Springer International Publishing AG
The registered company address is: Gewerbestrasse 11, 6330 Cham, Switzerland

Foreword

The number of joint replacement surgeries has been rising year after year due to advances in prosthesis design and implantation procedures, an aging population, and the general acceptance of this type of surgery. While the risk of infection in patients undergoing joint arthroplasty is low, the high and growing numbers of these procedures translate the low risk into a substantial and increasing burden of infection. Periprosthetic joint infections are associated with major patient morbidity, alongside substantial healthcare and societal costs. A better understanding of the risk factors, microbial etiologies, and pathogenesis of these infections will inform strategies to prevent, diagnose, and better manage them. The pathogenesis of periprosthetic joint infection has been shown to be related to antibiotic-tolerant biofilm bacteria. Making an accurate diagnosis as to the presence or absence of periprosthetic joint infection, and, if present, determining which microorganism(s) is (are) involved, is important for defining appropriate patient management. Overall, our application and understanding of diagnostics have improved over time, but there remain some open questions, alongside occasional puzzling culture-negative cases. Likewise, as a result of carefully performed studies and clinical observations, the management of periprosthetic joint infection has become more standardized, to the point where guidelines now exist.

I congratulate Dr. Trisha Peel on her timely and important book addressing critical issues related to periprosthetic joint infection.

Rochester, USA   Robin Patel

Preface

Prosthetic Joint Infections consist of five major parts describing the current approaches to the epidemiology, diagnosis, management, prevention, and summary recommendations for prosthetic joint infections. The editor is grateful to the expert contributors who have undertaken in-depth and comprehensive reviews for each topic, distilling the vast amount of literature into clear and concise overviews for each section. I sincerely thank all the coauthors for their dedication and contributions.

Melbourne, Victoria, Australia   Trisha Peel

Contents

Contributors

Natividad Benito Infectious Diseases Unit, Department of Internal Medicine, Hospital de la Santa Creu i Sant Pau, Universitat Autònoma de Barcelona, Barcelona, Spain

Jaime Esteban Department of Clinical Microbiology, IIS-Fundacion Jimenez Diaz, UAM, Madrid, Spain

Juan Pablo Horcajada Department of Infectious Diseases, Hospital del Mar, Barcelona, Spain

Courtney Ierano National Centre for Antimicrobial Stewardship, Royal Melbourne Hospital, Parkville, Victoria, Australia

Jaime Lora-Tamayo Department of Internal Medicine, Unit of Infectious Diseases, Hospital Universitario 12 de Octubre, Madrid, Spain

Oscar Murillo Department of Infectious Diseases, Hospital Universitari de Bellvitge, Institut d'Investigació Biomèdica de Bellvitge (IDIBELL), Universitat de Barcelona, Barcelona, Spain

Robin Patel Divisions of Clinical Microbiology and Infectious Diseases, Departments of Laboratory Medicine & Pathology and Medicine, Mayo Clinic, Rochester, MN, USA

Trisha Peel Department of Infectious Diseases, Monash University and Alfred Health, Melbourne, Victoria, Australia

Alba Ribera Department of Infectious Diseases, Hospital Universitari de Bellvitge, Barcelona, Spain

Alex Soriano Department of Infectious Diseases, Hospital Clínic, University of Barcelona, Barcelona, Spain

Ricardo Sousa Department of Orthopedics, Centro Hospitalar do Porto—Hospital Santo António, Porto, Portugal

Andrew J. Stewardson Department of Infectious Diseases, Monash University and Alfred Health, Melbourne, Victoria, Australia

Chapter 1
Introduction to Prosthetic Joint Infection

Trisha Peel

Total joint replacement surgery represents one of the highest volume medical interventions globally, contributing an estimated 0.65% to the world gross domestic product (GDP) [1]. The clinical and economic benefits of this surgery are undermined by the impact of prosthetic joint infection. These infections, while uncommon (1–3%), are associated with substantial patient morbidity, including the need for prolonged hospitalisation, repeat surgery, and antibiotic exposure [2].

Prosthetic joint infections are challenging to diagnose and treat, due to the unique behaviour of microorganisms when in contact with prosthetic material. In the presence of prosthetic material, such as a prosthetic joint replacement, the microorganisms undergo a change, transforming from the "free-living" or "planktonic" form that clinicians familiarly encounter in sepsis to the "stationary" or "sessile" form. In its sessile form, the microorganism develops complex archi-

T. Peel
Department of Infectious Diseases, Monash University
and Alfred Health, Melbourne, Victoria, Australia
e-mail: trisha.peel@monash.edu

© Springer International Publishing AG 2018
T. Peel (ed.), *Prosthetic Joint Infections*,
https://doi.org/10.1007/978-3-319-65250-4_1

1

tectural arrangements comprised of microorganisms within an extracellular "slime" or matrix: together, these microorganisms and the matrix constitute the "biofilm" [3, 4]. The microorganisms in the biofilm have a slower rate of turnover compared to the planktonic counterparts. The biofilm protects the microorganism against the host's immune responses and also impedes the activity of antimicrobial agents, therefore promoting the persistence of these infections [2–4]. The majority of modern-day laboratory techniques are optimised for the detection of planktonic microorganisms; therefore, detection of microorganisms in the biofilm is difficult [5]. As knowledge of biofilms increases, evidence for the optimal strategies to diagnose, treat, and prevent these infections is evolving, with a recent explosion in research and interest in these infections. This book provides a comprehensive review of the up-to-date evidence.

Through the development and maturation of national and international registries, the understanding of the current epidemiology of prosthetic joint infection continues to increase. These registries allow assessment of the incidence of infection and the capture of the changing ecology of causative microorganisms in an age of increasing antimicrobial resistance. Research has focused on the impact of patient-associated risk factors for infection, investigating the impact of potentially modifiable comorbidities such as obesity. In addition to increased understanding of the epidemiology of prosthetic joint infection, significant research has defined the impact on patient outcomes, such as pain and function, in addition to the economic impact of these infections on the healthcare system and society.

Previous efforts to diagnose prosthetic joint infection were limited to conventional laboratory culture techniques which lacked sensitivity and specificity. Over recent years, there have been significant advances in the approach to diagnosis of prosthetic joint infection. Among these is research examining strategies to improve conventional laboratory culture, including the introduction of sonication and the inoculation of periprosthetic tissue samples into blood culture bottles to improve the accuracy of diagnosis. There has been increased clarity around the optimal cut-off of currently applied inflammatory marker investigations such as C-reactive protein and synovial fluid properties, examining the differences in inflammatory marker profile in acute and chronic infections. New markers have been discovered and applied in a number of studies, of which alpha defensin, an antimicrobial peptide which is detected in synovial fluid samples in prosthetic joint infection, is the most promising marker to date.

Strategies in managing prosthetic joint infection have been reviewed by a number of centres, including by large multicentre research groups. There has been a concerted effort to define the optimal management of infections, guided by the chronicity of infection and the underlying causative microorganisms. Recent years have also seen an increased number of clinical trials, including randomised controlled trials, examining management aspects such as the ideal duration of antimicrobial therapy. Consensus guidelines, such as those produced by the Infectious Diseases Society of American and the International Consensus Group, have attempted to provide a uniform, evidence-informed approach to the management of prosthetic joint infection.

Finally, both the World Health Organization and the Centers for Diseases Control and Prevention have developed evidence-based guidelines for the prevention of surgical site infection, including prosthetic joint infection. These guidelines examine all aspects of the patient journey, including preoperative, intraoperative, and postoperative care. These evidence-based guidelines are important to ensure standardised approaches to patients undergoing surgery, to minimise the risk of postoperative infection and patient harm, and to ensure optimal outcomes for patients undergoing surgery.

Prosthetic joint surgery is one of the most successful surgeries performed in current day practice, with significant patient and health economics benefits. Knowledge of the best approaches to prevent these infections, one that includes understanding their underlying epidemiology, timely diagnosis, and optimal management, is critical to ensuring that the significant patient and societal benefits of this surgery continue to be realised.

References

1. Review on Antimicrobial Resistance. Antimicrobial resistance: tackling a crisis for the health and wealth of nations. London: UK Government and Wellcome Trust. 2014. https://amr-review.org/home.html. Accessed 30 Jun 2017.
2. Zimmerli W, Trampuz A, Ochsner PE. Prosthetic-joint infections. N Engl J Med. 2004;351(16):1645–54.
3. Costerton JW, Lewandowski Z, Caldwell DE, Korber DR, Lappin-Scott HM. Microbial biofilms. Annu Rev Microbiol. 1995;49:711–45.
4. Costerton JW. Bacterial biofilms: a common cause of persistent infections. Science. 1999;284(5418):1318–22.
5. Trampuz A, Piper KE, Jacobson MJ, Hanssen AD, Unni KK, Osmon DR, et al. Sonication of removed hip and knee prostheses for diagnosis of infection. N Engl J Med. 2007;357(7):654–63.

Chapter 2
Epidemiology of Prosthetic Joint Infection

Natividad Benito, Jaime Esteban, Juan Pablo Horcajada, Alba Ribera, Alex Soriano, and Ricardo Sousa

---

N. Benito (✉)
Infectious Diseases Unit, Department of Internal Medicine,
Hospital de la Santa Creu i Sant Pau, Universitat Autònoma de
Barcelona, Avenida Sant Antoni Maria Claret, 167, Barcelona
08025, Spain
e-mail: nbenito@santpau.cat

J. Esteban
Department of Clinical Microbiology, IIS-Fundacion Jimenez Diaz,
UAM, Madrid, Spain

J.P. Horcajada
Department of Infectious Diseases, Hospital del Mar,
Barcelona, Spain

A. Ribera
Department of Infectious Diseases, Hospital Universitari de
Bellvitge, Barcelona, Spain

A. Soriano
Department of Infectious Diseases, Hospital Clínic, University of
Barcelona, Barcelona, Spain

R. Sousa
Department of Orthopedics, Centro Hospitalar do Porto — Hospital
Santo António, Porto, Portugal

© Springer International Publishing AG 2018   5
T. Peel (ed.), *Prosthetic Joint Infections*,
https://doi.org/10.1007/978-3-319-65250-4_2

2.1   Incidence of Prosthetic Joint Infections

The joints that are most commonly replaced with a prosthetic implant involve total hip and knee arthroplasties. In addition to hip and knee replacements, shoulder, elbow and ankle arthroplasties are now available. Procedures to replace the wrist, temporomandibular, metacarpophalangeal and inter-phalangeal joints are less commonly performed. Virtually all extra-axial joints can be replaced with a prosthetic joint.

Total hip arthroplasty is indicated for patients who have failed previous treatment options for deteriorated hip joints but continue to have persistent debilitating pain and significant impairment in the activities of daily living. Displaced femoral neck fractures can also be treated with a prosthetic hip replacement. The indications for hip arthroplasty in the UK are osteoarthritis (93%), osteonecrosis (2%), femoral neck fracture (2%), developmental dysplasia of the hip (2%) and inflammatory arthritis (1%) [1]. The main indication for total knee arthroplasty is for the relief of pain and disability associated with osteoarthritis (primary or secondary) or inflammatory arthritis of the knee in patients who have failed nonoperative treatments [2]. Symptomatic osteoarthritis is the indication for surgery in more than 90% of patients, and its incidence is increasing because of an ageing population and the obesity epidemic in industrialized countries [3]. Osteoarthritis is one of the ten most disabling diseases in developed countries. Worldwide estimates indicate that 10% of men and 18% of women aged 60 years or older have symptomatic osteoarthritis, including moderate and severe forms [4]. Joint replacement surgery is considered the most effective intervention for severe hip and knee osteoarthritis, reducing pain and disability, restoring function and independence and improving the patient's quality of life [3]. While joint replacement surgery is mainly carried out in people aged 60 or more, it is increasingly performed in those who are younger [3].

An increasing number of joint replacements are being carried out in most of the industrialized countries worldwide, and the incidence of prosthesis implantation is expected to continue to rise. Procedures are referred to as either primary or revision arthroplasty, according to the number of times that a given joint is replaced. Primary arthroplasty is the first time that a native joint is replaced; revision arthroplasty is a second or subsequent surgical procedure performed when a joint replacement fails and some or all parts of the original prosthesis need to be changed. In 2009, a total of 284,000 primary total hip arthroplasties, 45,000 revision total hip arthroplasties, 619,000 primary total knee arthroplasties and 59,500 revision total knee arthroplasties were performed in the USA [5]. From 2009 to 2010, the total number of procedures increased by 6.0% for primary total hip arthroplasty, 6.1% for primary total knee arthroplasty, 10.8% for revision total hip arthroplasty and 13.5% for revision total knee arthroplasty [5]. The numbers of primary total hip and knee arthroplasty are projected to reach 572,000 and 3.48 million, respectively, by 2030 [6]. According to the Canadian Institute for Health Information, hip and knee arthroplasty rates increased by 16.5% and 21.5%, respectively, in the 5-year period from 2008 to 2013 [7]. The number of hip and knee replacements in most European countries has also increased in recent years, although rates between countries vary considerably [3] (Fig. 2.1). In the USA, primary shoulder and elbow

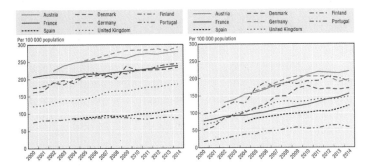

FIGURE 2.1 Trends in hip (*left*) and knee (*right*) replacement surgery, 2000–2014, selected European countries (OECD Health Statistics) (From OECD/EU [3], with permission)

arthroplasty procedures increased at annual rates of 6–13% from 1993 to 2007 [8]. The revision burden increased from approximately 4.5–7% [8].These numbers are anticipated to escalate further over the next few decades.

Most of the information about the incidence of prosthetic joint infection in the published literature has been hampered by methodological problems. These include a reliance on case series rather than well-designed cohort studies, the lack of explicit or standardized case definitions, incomplete case ascertainment, selection biases and, especially, differences in the length of follow-up [9]. Studies with longer follow-ups will report higher cumulative incidences (a percentage), even when the true incidence is low; failure to account for differences in length of follow-up between groups will lead to wrong conclusions [10]. Consequently, estimates of cumulative risk based on comparison should be made with caution unless the follow-up periods are the same. The denominator for the incidence rate is the prosthetic joint year.

The overall rate of prosthetic joint infections is highest in the first 2 years after surgery; the greatest risk of prosthetic joint infection occurs in the first 6 months after the operation and declines steadily after that [9, 11]; nevertheless, approximately 20–25% of all prosthetic joint infections occur after 2 years [11, 12]. According to a review by researchers from the Mayo Clinic in 2000, the combined incidence of total hip and knee arthroplasty infection was 5.9 (95% confidence interval [CI] 5.3–6.5) infections per 1000 joint years in the first 2 years following implantation and 2.3 (95% CI, 2.1–2.5) in years 2–10 [9]. The rates of late prosthetic joint infection (detected >2 years after the index operation) and of very late prosthetic joint infection (detected >5 years after the operation) for primary hip and knee replacements due to primary osteoarthritis performed between 1998 and 2009 were analysed from nationwide Finnish health registers [12]. The incidence rate of late prosthetic joint infection was 0.069% (95% CI, 0.061–0.078) per prosthesis year and was higher after knee replacement than after hip replacement (0.080 vs. 0.057). The rate of very late prosthetic joint infection was 0.051% (95% CI, 0.042–0.063) per prosthesis year, 0.058 for knees and 0.944 for hips [12]. The cumulative incidence of infection following primary hip or knee arthroplasty implanted between 1969 and 2007 was 0.5%, 0.8% and 1.4% at 1, 5 and 10 years, respectively, according to a population study in Olmsted County, Minnesota [13]. In the US Medicare population between 1997 and 2006, the incidence of prosthetic joint infection within 2 years of total knee arthroplasty was 1.55% and 0.46% between 2 and up to 10 years [11]. The higher early incidence of infection following implantation of a prosthesis followed by a decrease over time reflects the predominant effect of infection acquired during surgery, variable delays in symptom onset and diagnosis of infection after implantation and the decreasing susceptibility of prostheses to haematogenous seeding over time [9].

The establishment of national and international nosocomial surveillance networks has provided information on rates of surgical site infection after joint replacements. Fourteen European countries participate in the orthopaedic modules within the European Centre for Disease Prevention and Control surgical site infection surveillance network. The latest overall infection rates provided by the network for 2010–2011 were 0.7% for infection within 1 year of a knee replacement (95% confidence interval [CI] 0.7–0.8) (intercountry range 0.2–3.2%) and 1.0% for a hip replacement, including hip hemiarthroplasty (intercountry range 0.4–11.4%), with considerable variation in rates between countries [14]. A similar cumulative incidence of 0.9% (95% CI, 0.85–1.02) for prosthetic joint infections within 2 years of the index surgery was reported from Sweden's hip arthroplasty register between 2005 and 2008 [15]. European infection rates for hip and knee arthroplasty within the first year of the index surgery are in line with estimates from the National Healthcare Safety Network of the Centers for Disease Control and Prevention in the USA: 0.9% for hip and 1.3% for knee prosthesis from 2006 to 2008 [16]. Data from the Healthcare Infection Surveillance Western Australia shows that the incidence of infection for hip and knee arthroplasty was 1.4 (95% CI 1.2–1.6) and 1.4 (95% CI 1.2–1.5), respectively, in 2008–2013 [17]. A surveillance study of surgical site infections in patients undergoing surgical procedures from 2005 to 2010, conducted in 30 countries across 4 continents (America, Asia, Africa and Europe), showed infection rates within 1 year of a hip and knee replacement of 2.6% and 1.6%, respectively [18]. A recent review of several national surveillance networks in Europe and the USA reported considerable differences in data collection methods and data quality, mainly in follow-up and post-discharge surveillance [19]. In that review, the cumulative incidence of prosthetic joint infection after total hip arthroplasty ranged from 1.3% to 2.9% and from 0.7% to 3.7% following total knee arthroplasty [19]. Conventional surgical site infection surveillance focuses largely on infections detected at the hospital where the operation was performed. Infections diagnosed and treated at other healthcare facilities may consequently be missed by conventional surveillance, which can lead to varying degrees of underestimation of the infection rate [20]. In a US study, 17% of infections would have been missed using operative hospital surveillance alone [20]. In that study, when infections diagnosed at other centres were included, the cumulative incidence of infection in the year following surgery was 2.3% for total hip arthroplasty and 2% for total knee arthroplasty [20]. Other sources of information on the incidence of prosthetic joint infections are the national arthroplasty registers, although it has also been found that the rate of prosthetic joint infection may be underestimated also in arthroplasty registers [21, 22]. An important weakness of the arthroplasty registers is that they are not designed for registration of infections. In the Nordic arthroplasty registers, the surgeon decides—based on a subjective assessment— whether or not the revision/reoperation is due to an infection. Positive cultures will not be available until 2–7 days after surgery, but once the revision diagnosis is reported to the register, it is probably never changed [22].

In most, but not all, of the studies, the rate of infection for total knee arthroplasty is higher than for hip arthroplasty

[7, 9, 12, 16, 18]. The rate of surgical site infection is higher following hip hemiarthroplasty than total hip arthroplasty, ranging between 1.7% and 7.3% [23]. Hip hemiarthroplasty is the emergent surgical procedure indicated for displaced intracapsular femoral neck fractures, which are more frequent in the elderly population compared with total hip arthroplasty which is an elective procedure generally performed in younger people.

Some studies have reported an increasing incidence of prosthetic joint infections in hip and knee arthroplasties. Data extracted from the Nationwide Inpatient Sample in the USA showed that the incidence of prosthetic joint infection for hip arthroplasties increased from 1.99% (CI 95%, 1.78–2.21%) in 2001 to 2.18% (CI 95%, 1.97–2.39%) in 2009; after adjusting for other patient demographic factors, there was a significant year-to-year increase in the risk of hip infection over the study period [24]. The corresponding incidence rates for knee arthroplasties were 2.05% (CI 95%, 1.86–2.23%) in 2001 and 2.18% in 2009 (CI 95%, 1.99–2.37%). A more gradual but, nonetheless, significant increase in the risk of infection over time was found for knee compared to hip arthroplasty from 2001 to 2009 [24]. Similarly, the Nordic Arthroplasty Register Association (Denmark, Finland, Norway and Sweden) found an increase in cumulative 5-year revision rates due to infection in hip arthroplasties, rising from 0.46% (CI 95%, 0.42–0.50) during the period from 1995 to 1999 to 0.71% (CI 95%, 0.66–0.76) from 2005 to 2009 (6); the entire increase in risk of revision due to infection was within the first year of the primary surgery, and the risk increased in all four countries [25]. A population-based study, however, conducted in Olmsted County, Minnesota (USA), from 1969 to 2007, found no increase over the period of the study [13]. A recent study based on the Danish Hip Arthroplasty Register and several other national registers found that the relative risk of prosthetic joint infection in the year following primary total hip arthroplasty implantation did not increase over the 2005–2014 study period (the incidence was 0.53% [95% CI, 0.44–0.63] for 2005–2009 and 0.57% [95% CI, 0.49–0.67] for 2010–2014) [26]. In the study based on Finnish (nationwide) health registers of primary hip and knee replacements between 1998 and 2009, the incidence of late prosthetic joint infection (>2 years after the index operation) varied between 0.041% and 0.107% during the years of observation, with no temporal trend, while very late infections (>2 years after the index operation) increased significantly, from 0.026% in 2004 to 0.056% in 2010 [12]. By contrast, several national and international nosocomial surveillance networks have shown decreasing rates of surgical site infection after joint replacement in recent years [14, 17, 27, 28].

There is currently insufficient data to analyse the true incidence of arthroplasty infection at other anatomic locations, since the rates are based mainly on single-centre studies. After a shoulder arthroplasty, the rate of prosthetic infection appears to be similar to those for hip and knee prostheses, ranging from 0.98% to 1.3% in US series [29, 30]. The reported infection rate for elbow arthroplasty has been higher than for other joints: 3.3% in a systematic review [31]. The reasons for this may include an increased number of patients with rheumatoid arthritis (immunocompromised) receiving elbow arthroplasty and the fact that the elbow is a subcutaneous joint with a thin soft tissue envelope.

While it is still unclear whether the incidence of prosthetic joint infection is increasing, the absolute number of cases is growing. A further increase in the absolute number of arthroplasty infections is expected in the future, due to an increasing number of primary implantations carried out on a progressively elderly population with more associated comorbidities, the significant increase in the number of revision procedures, better methods of detection for the microbial biofilms involved in prosthetic joint infections, the increasing prevalence of microorganisms resistant to standard antibiotic prophylaxis and the accumulating number of arthroplasties that stay in place but remain at risk of infection during their implanted lifetime. Late infections occurring many years after prosthesis implantation may become more common, since the number of people living with some kind of joint arthroplasty is also increasing [12].

2.2   The Impact of Prosthetic Joint Infection

Prosthetic joint infections have a significant impact, not only on healthcare resources and economic costs but also on the morbidity, quality of life and mortality of patients. Research continues to quantify the impact of these infections.

2.2.1   Impact on Patient Mortality, Morbidity and Quality of Life

Prosthetic joint infection is widely depicted as a devastating complication with a potential impact on a patient's mortality and quality of life. Nonetheless, there is very little information in the literature about the quantity and quality of life of these patients.

Berend et al. [32] studied 205 infected total hip arthroplasties treated with a two-stage reimplantation protocol and found that, in spite of the high degree of infection control, there was a 48% mortality rate over the study period (1996–2009). Choi et al. [33] performed the first analysis of septic and non-septic revisions by investigating mortality rates in 93 patients after revision total hip arthroplasty matched to 93 control subjects. They found that the mortality rate in the septic group was 33% (31/93) and 22% (20/93) in the aseptic group at the 5- and 6-year follow-up, respectively. Although this difference was not statistically significant, the septic patients were younger and died 6 years earlier. The same authors performed a similar study focusing on 88 infected total knee arthroplasties and 88 controls [34]. The overall mortality rate following revision total knee arthroplasty was 10.7% after a median follow-up of 4 years but was 6 times higher after septic revision (18%–16/88) than after aseptic revision (3%–3/88) [34]. In order to determine the effect of prosthetic joint infection on mortality, Zmistowski et al. [35] compared the outcomes of 436 infected revisions with 2342 patients undergoing revision arthroplasty for aseptic failure. Prosthetic joint infection was associated with a fivefold increase in mortality, even after controlling for other variables. Mortality in the prosthetic joint infection cohort was 3.7% at 90 days, 10.6% at 1 year and 25.9% at the 5-year follow-up. These figures compare unfavourably with some of the most commonly dreaded cancers, such as female breast and uterus and male prostate cancer [36]. Of course, the increased risk of mortality is not only due directly to the adverse effect of infection and treatment but also to the fact that prosthetic joint infection often reflects a poorer health status. Nevertheless, these figures should raise awareness of the systemic impact of disease among those doctors involved in the management of these infections and of the need to concentrate on two highly interconnected dimensions when dealing with prosthetic joint infections: infection eradication and general health status.

There is extensive evidence to show that a successful total joint arthroplasty greatly increases the patient's quality of life in terms of function, pain and mobility, although surprisingly few studies in the literature about quality of life after prosthetic joint infections. Cahill et al. [37] were among the first to address this issue. They compared 62 uncomplicated total joint replacements and 34 cases of prosthetic joint infection, using a visual analogue scale for satisfaction, the Western Ontario and McMaster Universities Osteoarthritis Index (WOMAC), Assessment of Quality of Life (AQoL) and the Short-Form 36 (SF-36). They found that infection reduced patient satisfaction and seriously impaired functional health status and health-related quality of life, but provided no information about the influence of infection control on health status. Helwig et al. [38] analysed 58 patients with prosthetic joint infection, applying the Short-Form Health Survey 12 (SF-12) to evaluate physical and mental status according to the outcome of infection, but did not differentiate between those treated with debridement and implant retention and one- or two-stage revision protocols. Surprisingly, when they compared successful and unsuccessful therapies, they found no significant differences on either scale, suggesting that even after a good clinical outcome, patients remained physically and mentally limited. As expected, when the infected cohort was compared with the general German population, they found that physical status was significantly disadvantaged.

There is some debate about whether one- or two-stage exchange is the best surgical option for chronic prosthetic joint infection. The impact on quality of life would be a major consideration for deciding which is the most appropriate option, although it is not possible to draw definitive conclusions from the available data. One study analysed functional outcome after revision surgery for prosthetic hip infection, and two-stage exchange was the first therapeutic option for more severe infections and patients with more comorbidities [39]. Studies that compare different surgical options with similar patients or in clinical trials should include functional and quality-of-life analysis. At the same time, there is also little information about the functional outcomes of patients treated with open debridement and implant retention, a common surgical strategy for treating acute prosthetic joint infection. Aboltins et al. [40] prospectively collected pre-and post-arthroplasty data of 2134 total joint arthroplasty patients, in which there were 41 prosthetic joint infections. The main conclusion was that prosthetic joint infection cases treated with debridement and implant retention had a similar improvement from pre-arthroplasty to 12 months post-arthroplasty as patients without prosthetic joint infection in terms of quality of life, according to the SF-12 survey. The analysis did not evaluate the potential influence of aetiological microorganisms. Núñez et al. [41] evaluated 24 patients with acute knee prosthetic joint infection who underwent debridement and implant retention and were in remission after 12 months of follow-up. Their health-related quality of life was analysed using WOMAC and SF-36 at baseline (before knee replacement) and at 12 and 24 months after antibiotic treatment ceased. There was a significant improvement in all items from baseline to 48 months after the operation, except for patients infected with *Staphylococcus aureus* who had significantly worse outcomes, most especially in terms of stiffness and function on the WOMAC index and the

SF-36. Indeed, the only variables independently associated with worse outcomes were *S. aureus*, number of comorbidities and age. *S. aureus* is a virulent microorganism that causes severe soft tissue damage, which is potentially associated with a higher degree of fibrosis and scarring and would explain, at least in part, the worse functional outcomes.

Although more studies are needed to fully clarify the extent of the impact of prosthetic joint infection on a patient's quality of life, there is no doubt that it should be a concern for professionals involved in the management of these patients. According to the literature, debridement and implant retention for early postoperative prosthetic joint infection is associated with a similar quality of life to subjects who do not have infection except those caused by *S. aureus*. Early diagnosis and treatment would probably improve the results in such cases. Meanwhile, revision surgery for infection has been clearly associated with a significant deleterious impact on health-related quality of life.

2.2.2   Economic Impact

Prosthetic joint infection management represents a substantial economic burden for hospitals, healthcare systems and patients alike. Infection is consistently one of the leading causes of total joint revision surgery [42–45]. It is often the first or second most common indication for revision total knee arthroplasty [42, 44] and the third most common for revision total hip arthroplasty after aseptic loosening and dislocation [45]. It is also a leading cause of failure in other prostheses, specifically, shoulder, elbow and ankle prostheses [30].

The real cost of treating an infected joint is not easy to ascertain. It depends on many variables, such as the type of surgery, treatment, patient comorbidities and even bacterial factors, such as the antibiotic susceptibility profile. The full spectrum of economic impact includes not only the most commonly reported direct in-hospital costs but also direct outpatient costs (follow-up visits, rehabilitation, pharmacy), as well as indirect costs that are virtually impossible to gauge with any accuracy, such as loss of productivity or absence from work by the patient or his caregivers.

Kurtz et al. [24] included over 150,000 prosthetic joint infection cases and found that the average total hospital costs for infected hip revision were $72,700 US dollars (USD) in 2001, and $93,600 USD in 2009. The average charges for infected knee revision were $58,700 USD in 2001 and $74,900 USD in 2009. More recent studies from the USA included not only inpatient costs but also the cost of outpatient services. In 2014, Kapadia et al. [46] identified 21 infected total knee arthroplasties and matched them to 21 non-infected subjects who underwent uncomplicated primary surgery. Patients with prosthetic joint infection had significantly longer hospital stays, more readmissions and more clinic visits. The mean total episode cost (fixed and variable direct costs) for patients with surgical site infections was $116,383 USD (range, $44,416–$269,914), which was significantly higher than the mean $28,249 USD (range, $20,454–$47,957) in the matched group. Just recently, the same authors studied 16 consecutive infected total hip arthroplasties matched to 32 non-infected patients [47]. As before, the mean cost per episode was significantly higher in the infected group, $88,623 USD (range, $44,043–$158,202) than in the matched cohort, $25,659 USD (range, $13,595–$48,631).

The specific cost varies sharply from one setting to another, depending on the type of healthcare system and the corresponding economic standard. Fernandez-Fairen et al. [48] performed a systematic review of the literature and found significant disparities in absolute values between publications, depending on the country of origin. Nonetheless, the cost of a septic revision was consistently around 2–4 times more expensive than primary surgery and 1.5–3 times more expensive than aseptic revision surgery.

Cases of early postoperative and haematogenous prosthetic joint infection can be treated effectively with debridement and implant retention. The specific objective of an Australian study by Peel et al. [49] was to calculate the cost associated with this strategy. They focused on 21 prosthetic joint infections (12 total hip arthroplasties, 9 total knee arthroplasties) matched to 42 control patients with uneventful primary joint replacements. They included inpatient and also outpatient expenses, including readmissions, follow-up medical and nursing visits, medical imaging, pathology and pharmacy, including dispensed antibiotics. The total cost for patients with infection was $69,414 Australian dollars (AUD), compared with $22,085 AUD for the controls, with significant differences across almost all areas of patient care. The cost of an infection including the index operation and the costs of prosthetic joint infection management was 3.1 times that of an uneventful primary arthroplasty.

In summary, the economic cost of treating a case of prosthetic joint infection is two to four times higher than a primary replacement or aseptic revision.

More studies are needed that not only include a descriptive cost analysis but also take into account outcome measures, such as successful infection eradication, functional results and quality-of-life measurements after treatment. These cost benefit analyses will allow for more informed decision-making in all fields of prosthetic joint infection management. Prevention remains the best way to avoid the dire health-related and economic consequences of infection. Advances in the prevention of prosthetic joint infection will be needed to make an impact on the anticipated increase in the number of infections in the years to come.

2.3   Risk Factors

Several risk factors for the development of a prosthetic joint infection have been described, mainly derived from patients with total hip and knee arthroplasties. Some of the proposed risk factors should however be interpreted with caution because different studies used diverse methods or employed different classifications/scoring systems or focused on only one particular anatomic site [50]. Some studies have suggested that the risk factors could vary according to the particular anatomic joint [51]. Identifying the current risk factors that predispose patients to prosthetic joint infections after an arthroplasty will help the clinician establish strategies to prevent them. Risk factors for acquiring prosthetic joint infections can be categorized as patient characteristics, perioperative related factors and risk during bacteraemia [50].

2.3.1 Host Risk Factors

Nutritional status (mainly obesity), diabetes mellitus, rheumatic diseases and immunosuppressive therapy are among the most frequently reported risk factors for developing prosthetic joint infections [50, 52]. Smoking, coagulopathy, preoperative anaemia and previous joint surgery, mainly previous arthroplasty, have also been described as risk factors for prosthetic joint infection.

Obesity, defined as weight >20% above the ideal body weight or increased body mass index (BMI), has been associated with and increased risk of infection in several studies [52, 53]. Possible reasons include prolonged operative duration, increased allogenic blood transfusions and the presence of other comorbidities [54, 55]; however, obesity has remained an independent risk factor after adjustment for other covariates in some investigations [55]. In their study, Peel et al. described that for every 1 kg/m^2 increase in BMI, there was an associated 10% increase in the risk of prosthetic hip infection [51]. It was suggested that the association between obesity and hip arthroplasty could reflect an increase in postoperative dead space and the excellent medium for microbiological growth provided by necrotic fat [51]. Conversely, suboptimal preoperative nutrition with BMI <25 or malnutrition with serum albumin <34 g/L has also been associated with an increased risk of prosthetic joint infection [52, 54, 56, 57].

Diabetes mellitus is a risk factor for infection after general surgical and arthroplasty procedures [52, 58]. Moreover, Mraovic et al. observed that postoperative morning hyperglycaemia (blood glucose > 200 mg/dL) increased the risk of surgical site infection, even in patients without diabetes [59].

Patients with rheumatoid arthritis are at higher risk for developing prosthetic joint infections, with a relative risk increased approximately two- to fourfold, compared with that of patients without rheumatoid arthritis [9, 52, 60, 61]. This risk increases further in the context of revision arthroplasty or when there has been a previous prosthetic joint infection. It is often difficult to separate the relative contribution of the underlying illness, the accompanying comorbid conditions and the therapy with immunosuppressive or immunomodulating agents used with the patients [55]. New treatment approaches for patients with rheumatoid arthritis, including earlier use of disease-modifying antirheumatic drugs and the advent of biologic drugs, such as antitumour necrosis factor inhibitors, may have significantly increased the risk of prosthetic joint infections in these patients [61]. Until further data is available, the discontinuation of chronic treatment with these drugs should be assessed on a case-by-case basis before undergoing elective orthopaedic surgery. In their study, Peel et al. demonstrated that systemic corticosteroid therapy remained a predictor of infection when controlling for underlying comorbidity; this association may be mediated, at least in part, by impaired wound healing [51].

A systematic review found that smokers were substantially more likely to have postoperative complications following total knee or hip arthroplasty [62]. Current smokers undergoing knee or hip replacement had more often surgical site infections than never smokers. This is likely related to the negative effects associated with vasoconstriction on surgical wound healing [57].

Greenky et al. analysed 15,222 patients who underwent total joint arthroplasties from January 2000 to June 2007. A percentage of 19.6% presented with preoperative anaemia; prosthetic joint infection occurred more frequently in anaemic patients at an incidence of 4.3% compared with 2% in nonanaemic patients ($P < 0.01$) [63]. The multivariate model confirmed the risk of prosthetic joint infections to be two times higher in anaemic patients vs. nonanaemic patients.

A mean international normalized ratio (INR) greater than 1.5 has been found to be more prevalent in patients who developed postoperative wound complications (such as haematoma) and later prosthetic joint infections [64].

A history of prior arthroplasty on the index joint has consistently been recognized as a risk factor for prosthetic joint infection, increasing the risk of infection by up to eight times compared with patients with primary implantation [56, 60, 65]. The risk increases with the number of previous joint arthroplasties [60]. Prolonged operating times during revision surgery, the presence of unrecognized infection at the time of revision and abnormal surrounding soft tissue could be contributing factors.

S. aureus colonization increases the risk of *S. aureus* surgical site infections. The risk for these infections may be decreased by screening patients for nasal carriage of *S. aureus* and decolonizing carriers during the preoperative period [66, 67].

The presence of distant infections previous to the joint replacement has also been related to a higher risk of prosthetic joint infections, presumably due to transient bacteraemia from a distant infection site during this high-risk period [55]. Therefore, it has been recommended to screen for the presence of active infection elsewhere (such as urinary tract infection, respiratory tract infection, active skin infection, abscess or infected ulceration) prior to an elective prosthetic replacement. If asymptomatic pyuria or bacteriuria is associated with the development of prosthetic joint infections is not completely clear [68–70].

2.3.2   Perioperative Factors

It is considered that prosthetic joint infection is frequently acquired in the operating room during the arthroplasty procedure [57]. During arthroplasty, 50–67% of surgical gloves are estimated to be perforated, which is associated with increased infection rates. Handwashing, double gloving and changing gloves at regular intervals during the operation may be preventive strategies [71–73]. Human traffic in the operating room is associated with increased bacterial air counts, while opening and closing the theatre door disrupts the airflow around the patient, allowing microorganisms to enter the airspace around the surgical site [74]. Hypothermia could also facilitate prosthetic joint infection by inducing peripheral vasoconstriction with a substantial reduction of subcutaneous oxygen tension and directly inhibiting the inflammatory response [75]. The use of alcohol-based antiseptic skin preparations, combined with povidone or chlorhexidine, in the operating room [76], skin drapes and clipping hair immediately before surgery rather than the night before are associated with a reduced risk of surgical site infections [77]. A timely and appropriate perioperative antibiotic, according to the current guidelines for antimicrobial prophylaxis, is one of the most effective agents for the prevention of prosthetic joint infection [78]. It is recommended to administer the antimicrobial 1 h prior to surgical incision, with a repeat dose if the operation extends beyond 2 or 3 h, or if there is substantial blood loss [75, 77, 79].

Another independent risk factor predictive of prosthetic joint infection is the duration of the operation. The risk increases significantly when a procedure lasts more than 120 min, which is a reflection of more complex surgery, with prolonged surgical exposure and tissue damage during the procedure [80].

In essence, all wound complications (such as delayed healing, drainage or persistent dehiscence, haematoma, seroma) increase the risk of infection. Several authors have shown that developing a superficial surgical site infection not involving the prosthesis is a significant risk factor for prosthetic joint infection [60, 65, 81]. In Berbari et al.'s study, surgical site infection correlated with a 35.9-fold increase in the risk of infection in multivariate analysis [60]. Several authors have described local haematoma and wound discharge as risk factors for infection [51, 53, 56, 60]. One case-control study with 63 cases observed that drainage tube implants reduced the risk of subsequent prosthetic knee infections. However, previous studies have found that drainage tubes reduce haematoma formation; they have not shown a reduction in infection [51].

There are risk factors for prosthetic joint infections not primarily associated with the surgical procedure or wound healing. These include developing postoperative atrial fibrillation and myocardial infarction as independent risk factors. One plausible explanation is that all patients with serious cardiac complications receive aggressive anticoagulation with heparin or similar, which has been reported to be an independent risk factor for the development of prosthetic joint infection [53, 64]; also, the patients are generally older and sicker with pre-existing medical conditions that delay wound healing [53].

An association has been reported between allogeneic blood transfusion and infection related to the immunomodulation effect of the transfusion [82]; these patients are 2.1 times more likely to develop prosthetic joint infections, compared to those who do not receive a transfusion [53].

Longer hospital stays are another adjusted independent risk factor for infection. These patients are more likely to be exposed to nosocomial organisms that can lead later to prosthetic joint infection [53]. For this reason, it is important to avoid unnecessary stays in hospital before elective joint implantation.

2.3.3   Risk of Haematogenous Prosthetic Joint Infection

Finally, it is important to remark that an arthroplasty implant is at risk of infection not only in the immediate postoperative period but during their implanted lifetime due to the risk of bacteraemia. Nevertheless, the incidence of haematogenous seeding to a joint from a remote infection is low (0.1%) [83]. The situation is different in the case of *S. aureus*, where the rate of prosthetic joint infection after *S. aureus* bacteraemia is approximately 35% [84]. This means that if bacteraemia (mainly due to *S. aureus*) occurs, patients with uninfected prosthetic joints should be carefully monitored clinically for the development of prosthetic joint infection. In this situation, early diagnosis may avoid exchange of the prosthesis since infection can be cured with debridement and implant retention.

Along the same lines, the question of whether dental procedures alter the risk of prosthetic hip or knee infection has been actively debated in the last few decades. Recent case-control and cohort studies have finally concluded that the risk of infection in patients with prosthetic joints does not increase after dental procedures and specific antibiotic prophylaxis is not required [85, 86].

2.3.4   Risk Scores

The American Society of Anaesthesiologists (ASA) score is a widely used grading system for preoperative health of the surgical patients based in five classes. The ASA score has been associated with an increased risk of prosthetic joint infection in several studies [51–53].

The National Nosocomial Infections Surveillance (NNIS) System surgical score for identifying patients at a high risk of postoperative surgical site infection includes the ASA preoperative assessment score, the duration of the surgical procedure and surgical wound classification of each procedure (classification degree of microbial contamination of surgical wound at time of operation) [87]. The NNIS has been shown to be a better predictor of surgical site infection than individual components of the index. In one large case-control study, an NNIS score ≥1 was a significant risk factor for the development of prosthetic joint infections and an NNIS score of 2 correlated with a 5.2-fold increase in the probability of infection [60]. These findings remained in the multivariate analysis.

Two proposed Mayo prosthetic joint infection risk score models were developed using data from 339 cases and 339 controls of patients undergoing total hip or knee arthroplasty in the same period at a tertiary referral hospital; risk factors were detected using multivariable modelling [56]. The baseline Mayo prosthetic joint infection risk score included BMI (either high or low), a previous operation on the index joint, prior arthroplasty, immunosuppression, ASA score and procedure duration. This score has the potential to help identify high-risk individuals at the time of surgery. The 1-month-postsurgery score for risk of prosthetic joint infection contained the same variables, as well as postoperative wound drainage. The last score can be used in the postoperative period as an early workup in patients with early signs or symptoms suggestive of prosthetic joint infection. The two risk score models require external validation before they can be implemented in clinical practice [56].

2.4   Classification Schemes

Several classifications have been proposed for prosthetic joint infections. Their objective is to guide medical and surgical decisions in patients with prosthetic joint infections.

The Zimmerli classification divides prosthetic joint infections into three categories based on time to infection: early-, delayed- and late-onset infections. Early-onset infection occurs in the 3 months following arthroplasty. The microorganisms involved are usually more virulent and are inoculated into the surgical site during implant surgery. In this classification, delayed-onset infection occurs after 3 months and before 12 or 24 months. This type is usually caused by less virulent microorganisms that contaminate the surgical site during arthroplasty. Late infections occur between 1 and 2 years after arthroplasty and are considered to be mainly haematogenous in origin, although some are also caused by slow-growing bacteria acquired during the index surgery [88].

This classification is somewhat similar to an older one by Coventry et al., who defined three stages of prosthetic joint infection. Stage I is acute infection in the first 3 months after surgery; stage II is delayed infection occurring between 3 months and 2 years after arthroplasty and constant chronic pain after the operation; stage III is a haematogenous infection with a previously pain-free period [89].

Another important classification that is frequently used is the Tsukayama classification, which proposes four types of prosthetic joint infection [90]. Early postoperative infection occurs in the first month after arthroplasty. Late chronic infection occurs after this time and is generally associated with a more protracted clinical course. The third type is acute haematogenous infection, which is a late infection with a long, previously asymptomatic period and usually follows a more acute clinical course. The fourth type of prosthetic joint infection is a positive intraoperative culture, found in patients undergoing revision arthroplasty for presumed aseptic failure. This latter category and late chronic infection represent the same clinical scenario: a loosened prosthesis inserted months or years previously, although with the difference that the new prosthesis has already replaced the infected one at the time of diagnosis in the positive intraoperative culture category.

The Zimmerli and Tsukayama classifications are the most frequently used and are similar from a practical point of view. Except for the timing, a positive intraoperative culture and late chronic infection are equivalent to delayed infection in the Zimmerli classification. Tsukayama's haematogenous category is defined in the same way as Zimmerli's late category, except for the time limit, set at 2 years. In summary, early postoperative infections and haematogenous infections (Zimmerli's late type) can be regarded as acute infections, whereas Tsukayama's late chronic and Zimmerli's delayed prosthetic joint infections correspond to chronic infections.

Most teams use these classifications for deciding how to manage prosthetic joint infections. Patients with early postoperative and haematogenous infections are candidates for debridement and implant retention with prolonged antimicrobial therapy in an attempt to cure the infection without removing the implant. Late chronic and delayed infections are frequently managed with a two-stage implant exchange. This approach is based on the possibility of curing acute infections while biofilm is still immature and the difficulty of treating chronic infections with mature biofilms without removing the implant [91].

Other authors have added some useful considerations to prosthetic joint infection classifications. According to Garvin and Hanssen, acute prosthetic joint infections occur in the 4 weeks following surgery and late chronic prosthetic joint infections 4 weeks after surgery with an insidious clinical onset [92]. This insidious clinical onset is useful in daily practice for distinguishing between late chronic and late (acute) haematogenous prosthetic joint infections. Senneville et al. mainly considered the duration of the symptoms and attached less importance to timing with respect to surgery. Their classification proposes acute infection as one with <1 month of symptoms. Other infections with symptoms duration of >1 month are late infections [93].

As some studies on the subject of prosthesis retention have suggested, successful management of prosthetic joint infections depends on factors other than the time when infection occurs [94, 95]. Hence, factors such as the condition of the host, the appearance of the soft tissue around the prosthesis and the virulence of the microorganism causing the infection should be taken into account when deciding on the therapeutic attitude. McPherson et al. categorized prosthetic joint infections not only in terms of timing but also in terms of the systemic status of the host [96]. Their classification included early postoperative infection (stage I), haematogenous infection (stage II) and late chronic infection (stage III). Late chronic infection was considered when symptoms arose 4 weeks or more after the index arthroplasty. Patients were classified, on the basis of age, the presence of neutropenia and low CD4 cell count, as non-compromised (A), compromised (B) or significantly compromised (C). The infection site was also graded according to the presence of chronic infection, fistula, tissue loss and similar factors, as grade 1, 2 or 3 (uncompromised, compromised and significantly compromised, respectively). The use of this classification for the management of prosthetic joint infections has yielded different results in prognosis [96, 97].

2.4.1   Microbial Aetiology

Much of our current understanding of the microbial aetiology of prosthetic joint infections comes from studies that have limitations due to small sample size, single-centre experiences, lack of uniform or standardized definitions of infection and a variety of selection biases [9, 98]. Most studies have focused on specific categories of infection (mainly early-onset or chronic infections) or on infections treated with particular surgical strategies (largely debridement with retention of the prosthesis or two-stage exchange). Few studies have systematically described the full microbial aetiology of these infections [98].

A wide range of bacterial and fungal microorganisms can cause prosthetic joint infection (see Table 2.1). Aerobic Gram-positive cocci are the most common group of causative microorganisms (65–78%) [9, 55, 98], driven largely by infection with staphylococci, both coagulase-negative staphylococci and S. aureus, which account for 50–65% of all infections [55, 98]. S. aureus is a virulent pathogen and prosthetic joint infection by S. aureus typically presents with acute infection, although chronic infections have also been reported [99]. The group of microorganisms referred to as coagulase-negative staphylococci includes many species, with Staphylococcus epidermidis being the most frequently identified member of this group. Many are ubiquitous members of the skin microbiota. This group of organisms is the most frequent cause of chronic infection. Since much of the literature on prosthetic joint infection tends not to refer to individual species, the role of different species is unclear. Streptococcus and Enterococcus

TABLE 2.1 Microbiology results for culture-positive prosthetic joint infections (From Benito et al. [98], with permission)

Microorganism or microorganism group	Total no. (% [95%CI]) of culture-positive infections (*N* = 2288)
Aerobic Gram-positive cocci	*1777 (77.7 [75.9–79.4])*[a]
Coagulase-negative staphylococci (CNS)	905 (39.6 [37.5–41.6])[b]
Staphylococcus epidermidis	532 (23.3 [21.5–25])
S. lugdunensis	43 (1.9 [1.3–2.5])
S. capitis	35 (1.5 [1–2.1])
S. hominis	30 (1.3 [0.8–1.8])
S. warneri	19 (0.8 [0.3–1.2])
S. auricularis	15 (0.7 [0.3–1])
Other species of CNS	31 (1.4 [0.9–1.9])[c]
CNS without identification at species level	293 (12.8 [11.4–14.2])
Staphylococcus aureus	643 (28.1 [26.2–30])
Methicillin-resistant *S. aureus*	180 (7.9 [6.7–9])
Streptococcus species	207 (9 [7.9–10.2])[d]
S. agalactiae	65 (2.8 [2.1–3.5])
Viridans group streptococci without identification at species level	45 (2 [1.4–2.6])
S. mitis group	32 (1.4 [0.9–1.9])[e]
S. anginosus group	24 (1 [0.6–1.5])[f]
S. pyogenes	17 (0.7 [0.4–1.1])
S. pneumoniae	12 (0.5 [0.2–0.8])
S. dysgalactiae	10 (0.4 [0.1–0.7])
Other species of streptococci	6 (0.3 [0–0.5])[g]

(continued)

TABLE 2.1 (continued)

Microorganism or microorganism group	Total no. (% [95%CI]) of culture-positive infections ($N = 2288$)
Enterococcus species	182 (8 [6.8–9.1])[h]
E. faecalis	158 (6.9 [5.8–8])
E. faecium	13 (0.6 [0.2–0.9])
Other species of *Enterococcus*	6 (0.3 [0–0.5])[i]
Enterococcus spp. without identification to species level	6 (0.3 [0–0.5])
Other aerobic Gram-positive cocci	4 (0.2 [0–0.4])[j]
Aerobic Gram-negative bacilli (GNB)	***632 (27.6 [25.8–29.5])***[k]
Enterobacteriaceae	466 (20.4 [18.7–22])
Escherichia coli	208 (9.1 [7.9–10.3])
Proteus spp.	109 (4.8 [3.9–5.7])[l]
Enterobacter spp.	97 (4.2 [3.4–5.1])[m]
Klebsiella spp.	58 (2.5 [1.9–3.2])[n]
Morganella morganii	43 (1.9 [1.3–2.5])
Serratia marcescens	19 (0.8 [0.4–1.2])
Other *Enterobacteriaceae*	19 (0.8 [0.4–1.2])[o]
Non-fermenting GNB	218 (9.5 [8.3–10.8])
Pseudomonas spp.	202 (8.8 [7.6–10])[p]
Acinetobacter spp.	13 (0.6 [0.2–0.9])[q]
Ralstonia picketii	4 (0.2 [0–0.4])
Other non-fermenting GNB	6 (0.3 [0–0.5])[r]
Other Gram-negative bacilli	6 (0.3 [0–0.5])[s]

TABLE 2.1 (continued)

Microorganism or microorganism group	Total no. (% [95%CI]) of culture-positive infections (*N* = 2288)
Aerobic Gram-positive bacilli	***54 (2.4 [1.7–3])***
Corynebacterium species	50 (2.2 [1.6–2.8])
Corynebacterium striatum	17 (0.7 [0.4–1.1])
Other species of *Corynebacterium* spp.	12 (0.5 [0.2–0.8])[t]
Corynebacterium spp. without identification to species level	21 (0.9 [0.5–1.3])
Listeria monocytogenes	4 (0.2 [0–0.4])
Anaerobic bacteria	***156 (6.8 [5.8–7.9])***[u]
Anaerobic Gram-positive bacilli	117 (5.1 [4.2–6])[v]
Cutibacterium (formerly *Propionibacterium*) spp.	111 (4.9 [3.9–5.8])[w]
Clostridium spp.	7 (0.3 [0.1–0.6])[x]
Anaerobic Gram-positive cocci	33 (1.4 [0.9–2])[y]
Anaerobic Gram-negative bacilli	21 (0.9 [0.5–1.3])[z]
Bacteroides group	16 (0.7 [0.3–1.1])[aa]
Other anaerobic Gram-negative bacilli	8 (0.3 [0.1–0.6])[ab]
Anaerobic Gram-negative cocci	1[ac]
Mycobacterium species	***9 (0.4 [0.1–0.7])***[ad]
Fungi	***30 (1.3 [0.8–1.8])***
Candida spp.	27 (1.2 [0.7–1.6])[ae]
Other fungi	3[af]

(continued)

TABLE 2.1 (continued)

Unless stated otherwise, data are number (%) of patients with indicated characteristic

Files in **bold-italic** show the groups of microorganisms that include the microorganisms in the lines below; that is, they are the main big groups of microorganisms (1. Aerobic Gram-positive cocci 2. Aerobic gram-negative bacilli (GNB) 3. Aerobic gram-positive bacilli 4. Anaerobic bacteria 5. Mycobacterium species 6. Fungi)

Each group of these six big groups may include some subgroups of microorganisms. These subgroups cannot be identified in the current table, but they were marked in the original Table because they were placed at the left margin. These subgroups should be identified as the main subgroups belonging to the big groups. So, p.ex. 1. Aerobic Gram-positive cocci includes the next subgroups: 1.1. Coagulase-negative staphylococci (CNS) 1.2. Staphylococcus aureus 1.3. Streptococcus species 1.4. Enterococcus species; 2. Aerobic Gram-negative bacilli (GNB) comprises the next subgroups: 2.1. Enterobacteriaceae 2.2. Non-fermenting GNB, and so on

Each subgroup of microorganisms can include several microorganisms or sub-subgroup of microorganisms, that are identified in the original Table with indentation respect to the subgroup that they belong. P. ex. 1.1. Coagulase negative staphylococci (CNS) includes: Staphylococcus epidermidis, Staphylococcus lugdunensis

[a]More than one aerobic Gram-positive coccus was isolated in 232 out of 1777 (13.1%) episodes of prosthetic joint infection where these organisms were identified

[b]More than one species of coagulase-negative staphylococci was identified in 81 out of 905 (9%) episodes of prosthetic joint infection where these microorganisms were involved

[c]*Staphylococcus haemolyticus* 10, *S. simulans* 5, *S. saccharolyticus* 4, *S. schleiferi* 4, *S. cohnii* 3, *S. intermedius* 3, *S. lentus* 1, *S. saprophyticus* 1

[d]Two species of viridans streptococci were involved in four prosthetic joint infection cases

[e]*Streptococcus mitis* 18, *S. oralis* 7, *S. sanguis* 5, *S. parasanguis* 2

[f]*Streptococcus anginosus* 13, *S. intermedius* 6, *S. constellatus* 5

[g]*Streptococcus bovis* group 3, *S. salivarius* 2, nutritionally variant (deficient) streptococci 1

[h]*Enterococcus faecalis* and *E. faecium* were involved in one episode of prosthetic joint infection

[i]*Enterococcus gallinarum* 2, *E. hirae* 1, *E. durans* 1, *E. casseliflavus* 1, *E. avium* 1

[j]*Gemella morbillorum* 2, *Gemella haemolysans* 1, *Facklamia* sp. 1

TABLE 2.I (continued)

---

[k]More than one aerobic Gram-negative bacillus was isolated in 131 (20.7%) episodes of prosthetic joint infection due to these microorganisms

[l]*Proteus mirabilis* 101, *P. vulgaris* 2, *P. penneri* 2, *Proteus* spp. 4

[m]*Enterobacter cloacae* 82, *E. aerogenes* 11, *Enterobacter* sp. 4

[n]*Klebsiella pneumoniae* 51, *K. oxytoca* 6, *Klebsiella* sp. 1

[o]*Citrobacter* species 8 (*C. koseri* 6, *C. freundii* 2), *Providencia* species 7 (*P. stuartii* 6, *P. rettgeri* 1), *Salmonella* species 4

[p]*Pseudomonas aeruginosa* in all but five cases: *P. stutzeri P. stutzeri* and *P. putida* were identified in one case each and *Pseudomonas* spp. in three cases

[q]*Acinetobacter baumannii* 12, *A. calcoaceticus* 1

[r]*Comamonas* spp. 2, *Achromobacter* spp. 2, *Stenotrophomonas maltophilia* 1, *Ochrobactrum anthropi* 1

[s]Other Gram-negative bacilli include *Pasteurella multocida* 3, *Haemophilus* spp. 2, *Campylobacter fetus* 1

[t]*Corynebacterium diphtheriae* 6, *C. jeikeium* 4, *C. aquaticum* 1, *C. ulcerans* 1

[u]More than one anaerobic bacterium was involved in eight cases of prosthetic joint infection

[v]Two species of anaerobic Gram-positive bacilli were identified in one prosthetic joint infection

[w]*Cutibacterium acnes* 83, *C. avidum* 6, *Cutibacterium* without identification to species level 22

[x]*Clostridium perfringens* 3, *C. absonum* 1, *C. ramosum* 1, *C. septicum* 1, *C. sphenoides* 1

[y]*Finegoldia magna* 5, *Parvimonas micra* 5, *Peptostreptococcus anaerobius* 3, *Peptococcus niger* 4, *Peptostreptococcus* not identified to species level 15

[z]Two patients had more than one species of aerobic Gram-negative bacilli (three species in one case and two species in the other one)

[aa]*Bacteroides fragilis* 12, *B. stercoris* 2, *B. thetaiotaomicron* 1, *Bacteroides* sp. 1

[ab]*Prevotella* species 5 (*P. bivia* 2, *P. corporis* 1, *P. melaninogenica* 1, *P. buccae* 1), *Parabacteroides distasonis* 1, *Porphyromonas asaccharolytica* 1, *Fusobacterium* sp. 1

[ac]*Veillonella* sp.

[ad]*Mycobacterium tuberculosis* 5, *M. fortuitum* 4

[ae]*Candida albicans* 16, *C. parapsilosis* 6, *C. glabrata* 2, *C. tropicalis* 1, *C. famata* 1, *Candida* sp. 1

[af]*Aspergillus fumigatus* 2, *Scedosporium apiospermum* 1

species were involved in 9% and 8% of cases, respectively, in a recent large multicentre study [98]. Among the streptococci, *Streptococcus agalactiae* was the species most often isolated. More than 50% of *Enterococcus* species were involved in infections occurring in the first 90 days after prosthesis implantation, and more than 50% of cases were polymicrobial infections [100]. *Enterococcus faecalis* was isolated in more than 85% of enterococcal infections [98, 100]. In most past series, aerobic Gram-negative bacilli were implicated in less than 10% of cases of prosthetic joint infections [9, 55, 88]. Recently, however, studies in different geographical areas have reported higher frequencies of these pathogens, ranging from 17% to 42% [98, 101–106]. The percentage of *Enterobacteriaceae* appears to be increasing, and the most common species isolated (in descending order) are *Escherichia coli*, *Proteus* spp., *Enterobacter* spp. and *Klebsiella* spp. [98, 105]. Anaerobic bacteria were involved in 7% of all cases of prosthetic joint infection in the recent large multicentre study referred to above, with *Cutibacterium* spp. (formerly *Propionibacterium* spp.) being the most commonly identified anaerobic bacterium (5% of all infections) [98]. *Cutibacterium acnes* is a low-virulence microorganism, generally found in the skin microbiota and sebaceous glands. This microorganism can be inoculated at the time of surgery, but most infections have an indolent clinical course and are usually diagnosed months after prosthesis implantation. Less frequently isolated in prosthetic joint infections are aerobic Gram-positive bacilli, such as *Corynebacterium* spp. (2%), fungi (1%) and *Mycobacterium* spp. (<1%) [98]. Even though fungi are not commonly involved in prosthetic joint infections, the proportion of infections has significantly increased in recent years [98]. In decreasing order, the following species are involved in more than 80% of all prosthetic joint infections: *S. aureus, S. epidermidis, E. coli, Pseudomonas aeruginosa, E. faecalis and P. acnes* (it should be remembered that coagulase-negative staphylococci are not often identified to the species level, so that *S. epidermidis* may be the most common species) [98].

The threat of infection caused by multidrug-resistant organisms is increasing worldwide, yet little is known about their possible role in prosthetic joint infection. In one recent study, multidrug-resistant bacteria were involved in 14% of these infections, including methicillin-resistant *S. aureus* (8%) and multidrug-resistant Gram-negative bacilli (6%) [98]. The percentage of methicillin-resistant *S. aureus* varies in studies performed in different geographical areas [98, 103, 107]. Of particular concern are data that suggest an increase in the proportion of multidrug-resistant bacteria in recent years, mainly due to the increase in multidrug-resistant Gram-negative bacilli [98]. The significant (almost 18%) and increasing quinolone resistance found in a recent study is of greatest concern because ciprofloxacin is considered a cornerstone of the treatment of prosthetic joint infections caused by aerobic Gram-negative bacilli [108].

Most infections are monomicrobial; usually fewer than 20% of infections are polymicrobial [55, 98]. Aerobic Gram-negative bacilli, enterococci and *S. aureus* are, in decreasing order, the most commonly isolated microorganisms in polymicrobial infections [109]. Polymicrobial infections occur more often as early-onset infections, and they are also more frequent in infected hip hemiarthroplasty than total hip arthroplasty infections.

In 4–12% of cases, no microorganisms are detected [50, 110]. This is related to various factors, which include the use of preoperative antimicrobials; the definition of a positive culture result, whether a positive culture represents contamination; the method of obtaining and transferring culture samples to the laboratory; and the number and type of specimens obtained for microbiological diagnosis [55, 110]. The most important risk factor for culture-negative prosthetic joint infection is antecedent antimicrobial therapy.

Although the most common causative organisms of prosthetic joint infections overall are coagulase-negative staphylococci and *S. aureus*, there are significant differences depending on the category of infection [109]. Early infections are characterized by a preponderance of virulent pathogens (*S. aureus*, aerobic Gram-negative bacilli, mainly *Enterobacteriaceae* and *Pseudomonas aeruginosa*), multidrug-resistant organisms (methicillin-resistant *S. aureus* and multidrug-resistant

Gram-negative bacilli) and polymicrobial infections. Coagulase-negative staphylococci are the leading cause of chronic infections, while *S. aureus* is the most common isolate found in acute haematogenous infection. Gram-negative bacilli and *Enterococcus* spp. are significantly more often found in early postoperative infections than in other categories of infection, while *Streptococcus* spp. are more frequently found in haematogenous infections. The four most commonly involved species in each classification group in a large recent study were (1) chronic infections, *S. epidermidis* (33%), *S. aureus* (20%), coagulase-negative staphylococci not identified at the species level (17%) and *P. acnes* (5%); (2) early post-interventional infections, *S. aureus* (36%), S. epidermidis (16%), *E. coli* (15%) and *P. aeruginosa* (15%); and (3) acute haematogenous infections, *S. aureus* (39%), *E. coli* (13%), *S. agalactiae* (11%) and viridans group streptococci (5%) [98].

There are also differences in the relative frequency of the microorganism with respect to the infected joint, although staphylococci predominate in all types of prosthetic joint infection [55]. A large single-institution database from the Mayo Clinic suggests that hip arthroplasty patients have a lower frequency of *S. aureus* than coagulase-negative staphylococcal infection compared to patients with infected knee arthroplasty, where the frequency of the two types of staphylococci is similar [55]. Anaerobic bacteria, including *P. acnes*, seem to be more frequently identified in hip than in knee arthroplasty infections. Among hip arthroplasties, significant differences have been found in the aetiology of infected hemiarthroplasties (an urgent procedure for the treatment of femur fractures) and total hip arthroplasties (usually an elective procedure performed on patients with generative joint diseases) [111–113]. Patients with infected hip hemiarthroplasties are older, have more comorbidities and early infections than patients with infected total hip arthroplasties. Compared to total hip arthroplasty infections, hemiarthroplasty infections are characterized by a greater preponderance of Gram-negative bacilli, multidrug-resistant organisms and polymicrobial infections [111–113]. Shoulder arthroplasty infection is much more commonly caused by *C. acnes* than other prosthetic joint infections of other joint types. The notable presence of *C. acnes* may be related to the fact that it is prevalent on the skin of the upper body where there is a high density of sebaceous glands (a well-known habitat of this organism). Coagulase-negative staphylococci are also more frequently involved in shoulder infection than *S. aureus*. *S. aureus* and coagulase-negative staphylococci cause over three quarters of elbow arthroplasty infections [55].

In summary, most prosthetic joint infections are monomicrobial and caused by staphylococci; however, the rate of infection caused by aerobic Gram-negative bacilli seems to have increased in the last few years, as well as the proportion of multidrug-resistant infections, mainly due to the increase of resistant Gram-negative bacilli. These data suggest that empirical and specific antimicrobial therapy for prosthetic joint infections could become more challenging. Reassessing antimicrobial prophylaxis strategies and other preventive measures for patients undergoing joint replacement could be required [66, 104]. Identifying the risk factors for antimicrobial-resistant prosthetic joint infections may help prevent them.

2.5 Pathogenesis

In order for microorganisms to initiate an infection, they must be able to reach the implant, which is introduced into a sterile field in the body using an aseptic surgical procedure. Arguably, the most frequent way of reaching the implant is via the contamination of the prosthesis during implant surgery [55, 114, 115]. This is considered the probable origin of the majority of infections. Another mechanism is for infection to progress from a contiguous focus of infection. Infection of the surgical wound in the days following surgery could be the source of a deep infection. In some cases (especially knee surgery), it should be remembered that there is very little soft tissue between the prosthesis and the skin surface, so that a prosthesis-related infection can almost always be suspected when a surgical wound infection appears following knee implant surgery [116]. The contiguity mechanism can be the source of many acute infections and of a limited number of delayed ones. The last source of infection is haematogenous, when a micro-organism gains access to the implant from a distant focus during a bacteraemia episode. This mechanism is possibly the least frequent one, with haematogenous infections comprising around 10% of all prosthetic joint infections in most series [98].

Despite the different routes that microorganisms can take in order to reach the implant, the pathogenic process seems to be common in most of them, characterized, in terms of the theory put forward by A.G. Gristina, as "the race for the surface" [114]. According to this theory, the implantation of a prosthetic device initiates a race between bacteria and host cells to colonize the implant. If the bacteria win the race, they attach to the surface of the implant, start to multiply and prevent the host tissue from integrating with the device. If the host cells win, they cover the surface of the implant, so enhancing tissue integration and preventing bacterial attachment and subsequent infection. Differences between the host tissue and the characteristics of the bacteria can lead to different types of infection, but the bulk of the process is considered to be the same for all of them.

The process of bacterial adhesion is a complex one and can be divided into different stages according to the relationship established between the bacteria and the surface of the device [117, 118]. In the initial stages, long-range forces acting between the microorganism and the surface serve to bring them closer together; the forces are physical ones and include gravity, Van der Waals forces, other electrostatic interactions and Brownian movement. They act when the microorganisms are 100 μm away from the surface and so relatively weak; the bond that the microorganism establishes with the surface is thus not a strong one, and it is easy to detach the bacteria from the implant during this stage.

When bacteria come closer to the surface (10 μm or less), a new set of forces starts to act. These are strong forces of a chemical nature that establish a tight bond between the organism and the surface by means of ionic and covalent links. In this part of the process, the molecules present in the bacterial cell are extremely important, because they are the key to creating the bond mentioned above. These molecules, known as adhesins or MSCRAMMs (microbial surface components recognizing adhesive matrix molecules), vary depending on the bacterial species and so behave differently according to the material [119]. It should however be borne in mind that the surface of the implant is rapidly covered with host molecules (blood and extracellular fluid) during surgery. These host cell proteins act as receptors for most of the adhesins of the different microorganisms, such as the fimbriae or pili of Gram-negative organisms or the family of *Staphylococcus* proteins, which includes protein A, clumping factor A, fibronectin-binding protein A and others [120, 121]. However, microorganisms can also attach to uncovered device surfaces, as many in vitro studies have demonstrated, and differences between species can be found in this setting too [119, 122].

Once attached, the bacteria start to multiply and produce extracellular matrix, which is the main component of a biofilm. In some cases, bacteria produce toxins and other pathogenic factors that trigger an acute inflammatory response with polymorphonuclear leukocytes. In such cases, acute infection appears with a large number of planktonic organisms. However, beneath this process, a biofilm is developing, which may be the cause of delayed infection in the future [123].

Biofilm development is the most important pathogenic factor in infections related to biomaterials, including device-related osteoarticular infection [55, 115, 124]. A biofilm is a superstructure composed of microorganisms and extracellular matrix attached to a surface or associated with an interface, in which the organisms form complex communities and interact with each other, with metabolic processes that trigger differentiation into subpopulations of cells. Biofilm development starts when adhered bacteria start to multiply and produce extracellular matrix. This is the main component of biofilm and includes various proteins, glycopeptides, lipids, DNA and many other molecules in a species-specific composition, although water is the most abundant component in all cases. Extracellular matrix serves to protect its components from external aggression and is also the medium that allows sessile organisms to communicate with each other, a source of nutrients for the different cell populations inside the structure and the environment in which the various metabolic activities take place [124].

Bacteria are known to communicate with each other using quorum sensing [124]. This involves very small, species-specific molecules that can interact with other individual cells. When the cell density inside the biofilm is high enough (a quorum is reached), this communication becomes general rather than individual and the process of metabolic differentiation inside the structure is initiated, with the activation and deactivation of specific genes. This leads to the development of subpopulations of metabolically inactive organisms, actively multiplying ones, cells designed to detach from the structure in order to find new areas to colonize and the development of "persister" cells. "Persister" cells are of enormous medical interest because they behave like spores (metabolically inactive, extremely resistant to environmental aggressions), whose objective is biofilm survival, even if all other cells are destroyed.

Once it is fully established, the biofilm becomes an extremely important resistance factor against antibiotics and the host immune system by deploying the full range of its various mechanisms, including impermeability, metabolically inactive organisms and persister cells, activation and/or interchange with resistance genes and probably many others [125]. The phenotypic consequence of this is that increased concentration and effort is necessary to eradicate the bacteria inside the biofilms [126]. In many cases, this requires that the infected implant be physically removed in order to eliminate the biofilm [125].

Related to biofilm maturation is another pathogenic event that occurs in prosthetic joint infections: the ability of microorganisms to survive intracellularly. First suggested by Drancourt in 1993 [127], intracellular survival was recently demonstrated in experimental in vivo models [128]. The possible mechanism behind this phenomenon starts when sessile cells differentiate in order to detach themselves from the mature biofilm. Various nonprofessional phagocytes, such as osteoblasts, fibroblasts, epithelial cells and so on, are able to phagocytize these bacteria, which are nevertheless able to survive within the phagocyte. This process has been studied in greater detail for "small colony variants" (SCV) of S. aureus

[129, 130]. These strains are able to survive intracellularly without destroying the cell because they lack some of the enzymes responsible for cell lysis when usual strains of *S. aureus* are internalized [130]. In those cases where a biofilm is physically removed, the intracellular cells can be regarded as a bacterial reservoir. In this situation, the intracellular organisms could be the source of a new colony on the new prosthesis, with a new biofilm and the development of a new infection (Fig. 2.2).

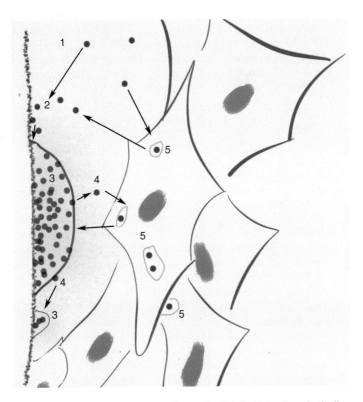

FIGURE 2.2 Pathogenic process of prosthetic joint infections including adherence steps, biofilm development and intracellular bacteria, with the potential relationships between them. 1 Bacterial adherence (weak forces), 2 bacterial adherence (strong forces), 3 biofilm development (bacterial multiplication and production of extracellular matrix); 4 biofilm development (bacterial detachment); 5 intracellular bacteria

The pathogenesis of prosthetic joint infections is a complex procedure that needs to be taken into account in order to establish proper therapy for the patient, because of the important implications of these phenomena for the outcome of the patient.

References

1. Pivec R, Johnson AJ, Mears SC, Mont MA. Hip arthroplasty. Lancet. 2012;380(9855):1768–77.
2. Carr AJ, Robertsson O, Graves S, Price AJ, Arden NK, Judge A, Beard DJ. Knee replacement. Lancet. 2012;379(9823):1331–40.
3. OECD/EU. Health at a glance: Europe 2016: state of health in the EU cycle. Paris: OECD; 2016. https://doi.org/10.1787/9789264265592-en. Accessed 9 Jan 2017.
4. World Health Organization. Chronic diseases and health promotion: chronic rheumatic conditions. 2017. http://www.who.int/chp/topics/rheumatic/en/. Accessed 2 Jan 2017.
5. Kurtz SM, Ong KL, Lau E, Bozic KJ. Impact of the economic downturn on total joint replacement demand in the United States. J Bone Joint Surg Am. 2014;96(8):624–30.
6. Kurtz S, Ong K, Lau E, Mowat F, Halpern M. Projections of primary and revision hip and knee arthroplasty in the United States from 2005 to 2030. J Bone Joint Surg Am. 2007;89(4):780–5.
7. Rennert-May E, Bush K, Vickers D, Smith S. Use of a provincial surveillance system to characterize postoperative surgical site infections after primary hip and knee arthroplasty in Alberta, Canada. Am J Infect Control. 2016;44(11):1310–4.
8. Day JS, Lau E, Ong KL, Williams GR, Ramsey ML, Kurtz SM. Prevalence and projections of total shoulder and elbow arthroplasty in the United States to 2015. J Shoulder Elb Surg. 2010;19(8):1115–20.
9. Steckelberg JM, Osmon DR. Prosthetic joint infections. In: Waldvogel FA, Bisno AL, editors. Infections associated with indwelling medical devices. 3rd ed. Washington: American Society of Microbiology; 2000. p. 173–209.
10. Lidwell OM. Apparent improvement in the outcome of hip or knee-joint replacement operations over the period of a prospective study. J Hyg. 1986;97(3):501–2.

11. Kurtz SM, Ong KL, Lau E, Bozic KJ, Berry D, Parvizi J. Prosthetic joint infection risk after TKA in the Medicare population. Clin Orthop Relat Res. 2010;468(1):52–6.

12. Huotari K, Peltola M, Jämsen E. The incidence of late prosthetic joint infections. Acta Orthop. 2015;86:321–5.

13. Tsaras G, Osmon DR, Mabry T, Lahr B, St Sauveur J, Yawn B, et al. Incidence, secular trends, and outcomes of prosthetic joint infection: a population-based study, Olmsted county, Minnesota, 1969-2007. Infect Control Hosp Epidemiol. 2012;33(12):1207–12.

14. European Centre for Disease Prevention and Control. Surveillance of surgical site infections in Europe 2010–2011. Stockholm: ECDC. 2013. Accessed 3 Feb 2017.

15. Lindgren V, Gordon M, Wretenberg P, Kärrholm J, Garellick G. Deep infection after total hip replacement: a method for national incidence surveillance. Infect Control Hosp Epidemiol. 2014;35(12):1491–6.

16. Edwards JR, Peterson KD, Mu Y, Banerjee S, Allen-Bridson K, Morrell G, et al. National Healthcare Safety Network (NHSN) report: data summary for 2006 through 2008, issued December 2009. Am J Infect Control. 2009;37(10):783–805.

17. McCann R, Peterson A, Tempone S. Healthcare associated infection unit. Healthcare infection surveillance Western Australia annual report 2012–2013. Perth: Department of Health Western Australia. 2013. http://www.public.health.wa.gov.au/cproot/5796/2/hiswa-2012-13-ar-final.pdf. Accessed 6 Jan 2017.

18. Rosenthal VD, Richtmann R, Singh S, Apisarnthanarak A, Kübler A, Viet-Hung N, et al. International nosocomial infection control consortium, surgical site infections, international nosocomial infection control consortium (INICC) report, data summary of 30 countries, 2005–2010. Infect Control Hosp Epidemiol. 2013;34(6):597–604.

19. Grammatico-Guillon L, Rusch E, Astagneau P. Surveillance of prosthetic joint infections: international overview and new insights for hospital databases. J Hosp Infect. 2015;89(2):90–8.

20. Yokoe DS, Avery TR, Platt R, Huang SS. Reporting surgical site infections following total hip and knee arthroplasty: impact of limiting surveillance to the operative hospital. Clin Infect Dis. 2013;57(9):1282–8.

21. Gundtoft PH, Overgaard S, Schønheyder HC, Møller JK, Kjærsgaard-Andersen P, Pedersen AB. The "true" incidence of

surgically treated deep prosthetic joint infection after 32,896 primary total hip arthroplasties: a prospective cohort study. Acta Orthop. 2015;86(3):326–34.

22. Witso E. The rate of prosthetic joint infection is underestimated in the arthroplasty registers. Acta Orthop. 2015;86(3):277–8.

23. Noailles T, Brulefert K, Chalopin A, Longis PM, Gouin F. What are the risk factors for post-operative infection after hip hemiarthroplasty? Systematic review of literature. Int Orthop. 2016;40(9):1843–8.

24. Kurtz SM, Lau E, Watson H, Schmier JK, Parvizi J. Economic burden of periprosthetic joint infection in the United States. J Arthroplasty. 2012;27(8 Suppl):61–65.e1.

25. Dale H, Fenstad AM, Hallan G, Havelin LI, Furnes O, Overgaard S, et al. Increasing risk of prosthetic joint infection after total hip arthroplasty. Acta Orthop. 2012;83(5):449–58.

26. Gundtoft PH, Pedersen AB, Schønheyder HC, Møller JK, Overgaard S. One-year incidence of prosthetic joint infection in total hip arthroplasty: a cohort study with linkage of the Danish hip Arthroplasty register and Danish microbiology databases. Osteoarthr Cartil. 2017;25:685. https://doi.org/10.1016/j.joca.2016.12.010.

27. State of Victoria Department of Health. Healthcare-associated infection in Victoria: surveillance report for 2010–11 and 2011–12. Melbourne: Victorian Government. 2014. https://www.vicniss.org.au/media/1020/vicnissannualreport2010-112011-12.pdf.

28. Choi HJ, Adiyani L, Sung J, Choi JY, Kim HB, Kim YK, et al. Korean nosocomial infections Surveillance system (KONIS). Five-year decreased incidence of surgical site infections following gastrectomy and prosthetic joint replacement surgery through active surveillance by the Korean nosocomial infection surveillance system. J Hosp Infect. 2016;93(4):339–46.

29. Singh JA, Sperling JW, Schleck C, Harmsen W, Cofield RH. Periprosthetic infections after shoulder hemiarthroplasty. J Shoulder Elb Surg. 2012;21(10):1304–9.

30. Padegimas EM, Maltenfort M, Ramsey ML, Williams GR, Parvizi J, Namdari S. Periprosthetic shoulder infection in the United States: incidence and economic burden. J Shoulder Elb Surg. 2015;24(5):741–6.

31. Voloshin I, Schippert DW, Kakar S, Kaye EK, Morrey BF. Complications of total elbow replacement: a systematic review. J Shoulder Elb Surg. 2011;20(1):158–68.

32. Berend KR, Lombardi A, Morris MJ, Bergeson AG, Adams JB, Sneller MA, et al. Two-stage treatment of hip periprosthetic joint infection is associated with a high rate of infection control but high mortality. Clin Orthop Relat Res. 2013;471(2):510–8.

33. Choi H-R, Beecher B, Bedair H. Mortality after septic versus aseptic revision total hip arthroplasty: a matched-cohort study. J Arthroplast. 2013;28(8 Suppl):56–8.

34. Choi HR, Bedair H. Mortality following revision total knee arthroplasty: a matched cohort study of septic versus aseptic revisions. J Arthroplast. 2014;29(6):1216–8.

35. Zmistowski B, Karam JA, Durinka JB, Casper DS, Parvizi J. Periprosthetic joint infection increases the risk of one-year mortality. J Bone Joint Surg Am. 2013;95(24):2177–84.

36. Howlader N, Noone AM, Krapcho M, Miller D, Bishop K, Altekruse SF, et al. SEER cancer statistics review, 1975–2013. Bethesda MD, USA: National Cancer Institute. http://seer.cancer.gov/csr/1975_2013/, based on November 2015 SEER data submission, posted to the SEER web site, April 2016. Accessed 12 Jan 2017.

37. Cahill JL, Shadbolt B, Scarvell JM, Smith PN. Quality of life after infection in total joint replacement. J Orthop Surg (Hong Kong). 2008;16(1):58–65.

38. Helwig P, Morlock J, Oberst M, Hauschild O, Hübner J, Borde J, et al. Periprosthetic joint infection—effect on quality of life. Int Orthop. 2014;38(5):1077–81.

39. De Man FHR, Sendi P, Zimmerli W, Maurer TB, Ochsner PE, Ilchmann T. Infectiological, functional, and radiographic outcome after revision for prosthetic hip infection according to a strict algorithm. Acta Orthop. 2011;82(1):27–34.

40. Aboltins C, Dowsey M, Peel T, Lim WK, Choong P. Good quality of life outcomes after treatment of prosthetic joint infection with debridement and prosthesis retention. J Orthop Res. 2016;34(5):898–902.

41. Núñez M, Vilchez Cavazos F, Núñez Juarez E, Martinez-Pastor JC, Maculé Beneyto F, Suso S, Soriano VA. Measuring outcomes: pain and quality of life 48 months after acute postoperative total knee prosthetic joint infection. Pain Pract. 2015;15(7):610–7.

42. Kamath AF, Ong KL, Lau E, Chan V, Vail TP, Rubash HE, Berry DJ, Bozic KJ. Quantifying the burden of revision total joint arthroplasty for periprosthetic infection. J Arthroplast. 2015;30(9):1492–7.

43. Le DH, Goodman SB, Maloney WJ, Huddleston JI. Current modes of failure in TKA: infection, instability, and stiffness predominate. Clin Orthop Relat Res. 2014;472(7):2197–200.
44. Sharkey PF, Lichstein PM, Shen C, Tokarski AT, Parvizi J. Why are total knee arthroplasties failing today—has anything changed after 10 years? J Arthroplast. 2014;29(9):1774–8.
45. Norwegian National Advisory Unit on Arthroplasty and Hip Fractures. Report June 2015. Bergen: Helse Bergen HF, Department of Orthopaedic Surgery, Haukeland University Hospital. 2015. http://nrlweb.ihelse.net/Rapporter/Report2015_english.pdf. Accessed 15 Jan 2017.
46. Kapadia BH, McElroy MJ, Issa K, Johnson AJ, Bozic KJ, Mont MA. The economic impact of periprosthetic infections following total knee arthroplasty at a specialized tertiary-care center. J Arthroplast. 2014;29(5):929–32.
47. Kapadia BH, Banerjee S, Cherian JJ, Bozic KJ, Mont MA. The economic impact of periprosthetic infections after total hip arthroplasty at a specialized tertiary-care center. J Arthroplast. 2016;31(7):1422–6.
48. Fernandez-Fairen M, Torres A, Menzie A, Hernandez-Vaquero D, Fernandez-Carreira JM, Murcia-Mazon A, et al. Economical analysis on prophylaxis, diagnosis, and treatment of periprosthetic infections. Open Orthop J. 2013;7:227–42.
49. Peel TN, Dowsey MM, Buising KL, Liew D, Choong PF. Cost analysis of debridement and retention for management of prosthetic joint infection. Clin Microbiol Infect. 2013;19(2):181–6.
50. Zimmerli W, Sendi P. Orthopedic implant-associated infections. In: Bennett JE, Dolin R, Blaser MJ, editors. Mandell, Douglas, and Bennett's principles and practice of infectious diseases. 8th ed. New York: Elsevier Sanders; 2015. p. 1328–40.
51. Peel TN, Dowsey MM, Daffy JR, Stanley PA, Choong PF, Buising KL. Risk factors for prosthetic hip and knee infections according to arthroplasty site. J Hosp Infect. 2011;79(2):129–33.
52. Zhu Y, Zhang F, Chen W, Liu S, Zhang Q, Zhang Y. Risk factors for periprosthetic joint infection after total joint arthroplasty: a systematic review and meta-analysis. J Hosp Infect. 2015;89(2):82–9.
53. Pulido L, Ghanem E, Joshi A, Purtill JJ, Parvizi J. Periprosthetic joint infection: the incidence, timing, and predisposing factors. Clin Orthop Relat Res. 2008;466(7):1710–5.
54. Kapadia BH, Berg RA, Daley JA, Fritz J, Bhave A, Mont MA. Periprosthetic joint infection. Lancet. 2016;387(100016):386–94.

55. Tande AJ, Patel R. Prosthetic joint infection. Clin Microbiol Rev. 2014;27(2):302–45.

56. Berbari EF, Osmon DR, Lahr B, Eckel-Passow JE, Tsaras G, Hanssen AD, et al. The Mayo prosthetic joint infection risk score: implication for surgical site infection reporting and risk stratification. Infect Control Hosp Epidemiol. 2012;33(8):774–81.

57. Marculescu CE, Mabry T, Berbari EF. Prevention of surgical site infections in joint replacement surgery. Surg Infect. 2016;17(2):152–7.

58. Namba RS, Inacio MCS, Paxton EW. Risk factors associated with deep surgical site infections after primary total knee arthroplasty: an analysis of 56,216 knees. J Bone Joint Surg Am. 2013;95(9):775–82.

59. Mraovic B, Suh D, Jacovides C, Parvizi J. Perioperative hyperglycemia and postoperative infection after lower limb arthroplasty. J Diabetes Sci Technol. 2011;5(2):412–8.

60. Berbari EF, Hanssen AD, Duffy MC, Steckelberg JM, Ilstrup DM, Harmsen WS, Osmon DR. Risk factors for prosthetic joint infection: case-control study. Clin Infect Dis. 1998;27(5):1247–54.

61. Bongartz T, Halligan CS, Osmon DR, Reinalda MS, Bamlet WR, Crowson CS. Incidence and risk factors of prosthetic joint infection after total hip or knee replacement in patients with rheumatoid arthritis. Arthritis Rheum. 2008;59(12):1713–20.

62. Singh JA. Smoking and outcomes after knee and hip arthroplasty: a systematic review. J Rheumatol. 2011;38(9):1824–34.

63. Greenky M, Gandhi K, Pulido L, Restrepo C, Parvizi J. Preoperative anemia in total joint arthroplasty: is it associated with periprosthetic joint infection? Clin Orthop Relat Res. 2012;470(10):2695–701.

64. Parvizi J, Ghanem E, Joshi A, Sharkey PF, Hozack WJ, Rothman RH. Does "excessive" anticoagulation predispose to periprosthetic infection? J Arthroplast. 2007;22(5 Suppl 2):24–8.

65. Poss R, Thornhill TS, Ewald FC, Thomas WH, Batte NJ, Sledge CB. Factors influencing the incidence and outcome of infection following total joint arthroplasty. Clin Orthop Relat Res. 1984;182:117–26.

66. Schweizer ML, Chiang HY, Septimus E, Moody J, Braun B, Hafner J, et al. Association of a bundled intervention with surgical site infections among patients undergoing cardiac, hip, or knee surgery. JAMA. 2015;313(21):2162–71.

67. Chen AF, Heyl AE, Xu PZ, Rao N, Klatt BA. Preoperative decolonization effective at reducing staphylococcal colonization in total joint arthroplasty patients. J Arthroplast. 2013;28(8 Suppl):18–20.

68. Gou W, Chen J, Jia Y, Wang Y. Preoperative asymptomatic leucocyturia and early prosthetic joint infections in patients undergoing joint arthroplasty. J Arthroplast. 2014;29(3):473–6.

69. Cordero-Ampuero J, González-Fernández E, Martínez-Vélez D, Esteban J. Are antibiotics necessary in hip arthroplasty with asymptomatic bacteriuria? Seeding risk with/without treatment. Clin Orthop Relat Res. 2013;471(12):3822–9.

70. Sousa R, Muñoz-Mahamud E, Quayle J, Dias da Costa L, Casals C, Scott P. Is asymptomatic bacteriuria a risk factor for prosthetic joint infection? Clin Infect Dis. 2014;59(1):41–7.

71. Adeli B, Parvizi J. Strategies for the prevention of periprosthetic joint infection. J Bone Joint Surg Br. 2012;94(11 Suppl A):42–6.

72. Al-Maiyah M, Bajwa A, Mackenney P, Port A, Gregg PJ, Hill D, Finn P. Glove perforation and contamination in primary total hip arthroplasty. J Bone Joint Surg Br. 2005;87(4):556–9.

73. Tanner J, Parkinson H. Double gloving to reduce surgical cross-infection. Cochrane Database Syst Rev. 2006;(3):CD003087.

74. Panahi P, Stroh M, Casper DS, Parvizi J, Austin MS. Operating room traffic is a major concern during total joint arthroplasty hip. Clin Orthop Relat Res. 2012;470(10):2690–4.

75. Meehan J, Jamali AA, Nguyen H. Prophylactic antibiotics in hip and knee arthroplasty. J Bone Joint Surg Am. 2009;91(10):2480–90.

76. Larson E. Guideline for use of topical antimicrobial agents. Am J Infect Control. 1988;16(6):253–66.

77. Mangram AJ, Horan TC, Pearson ML, Silver LC, Jarvis WR. Guideline for prevention of surgical site infection, 1999. Hospital infection control practices advisory committee. Infect Control Hosp Epidemiol. 1999;20(4):250–78. quiz 279-80

78. Bratzler DWW, Houck PM, Surgical Infection Prevention Guidelines Writers Workgroup, et al. Antimicrobial prophylaxis for surgery: an advisory statement from the national surgical infection prevention project. Clin Infect Dis. 2004;38(12):1706–15. Review

79. Prokuski L. Prophylactic antibiotics in orthopaedic surgery. J Am Acad Orthop Surg. 2008;16(5):283–93.

80. Ridgeway S, Wilson J, Charlet A, Kafatos G, Pearson A, Coello R. Infection of the surgical site after arthroplasty of the hip. J Bone Joint Surg Br. 2005;87(6):844–50.

81. Wymenga AB, van Horn JR, Theeuwes A, Muytjens HL, Slooff TJ. Perioperative factors associated with septic arthritis after arthroplasty. Prospective multicenter study of 362 knee and 2,651 hip operations. Acta Orthop Scand. 1992;63(6):665–71.

82. Raghavan M, Marik PE. Anemia, allogenic blood transfusion, and immunomodulation in the critically ill. Chest. 2005;127(1):295–307.

83. Uçkay I, Lübbeke A, Emonet S, Tovmirzaeva L, Stern R, Ferry T, et al. Low incidence of haematogenous seeding to total hip and knee prostheses in patients with remote infections. J Infect. 2009;59(5):337–45.

84. Sendi P, Banderet F, Graber P, Zimmerli W. Periprosthetic joint infection following Staphylococcus aureus bacteremia. J Infect. 2011;63(1):17–22.

85. Kao FC, Hsu YC, Chen WH, Lin JN, Lo YY, Tu YK. Prosthetic joint infection following invasive dental procedures and antibiotic prophylaxis in patients with hip or knee arthroplasty. Infect Control Hosp Epidemiol. 2016;38(2):154–61.

86. Berbari EF, Osmon DR, Carr A, Hanssen AD, Baddour LM, Greene D, et al. Dental procedures as risk factors for prosthetic hip or knee infection: a hospital-based prospective case-control study. Clin Infect Dis. 2010;50(6):8–16.

87. National nosocomial infections surveillance (NNIS) report, data summary from October 1986–April 1996, issued May 1996. A report from the National nosocomial infections surveillance (NNIS) System. Am J Infect Control. 1996; 24(5):380–8.

88. Zimmerli W, Trampuz A, Ochsner PE. Prosthetic-joint infections. N Engl J Med. 2004;351(16):1645–54.

89. Coventry MB. Treatment of infections occurring in total hip surgery. Orthop Clin North Am. 1975;6(4):991–1003.

90. Tsukayama DT, Estrada R, Gustilo RB. Infection after total hip arthroplasty. A study of the treatment of one hundred and six infections. J Bone Joint Surg Am. 1996;78(4):512–23.

91. Osmon DR, Berbari EF, Berendt AR, Lew D, Zimmerli W, Steckelberg JM, et al. Diagnosis and management of prosthetic joint infection: clinical practice guidelines by the Infectious Diseases Society of America. Clin Infect Dis. 2013;56(1):e1–e25.

92. Garvin KL, Hanssen AD. Infection after total hip arthroplasty. Past, present, and future. J Bone Joint Surg Am. 1995;77(10):1576–88.

93. Senneville E, Joulie D, Legout L, Valette M, Dezèque H, Beltrand E, et al. Outcome and predictors of treatment failure in total hip/knee prosthetic joint infections due to Staphylococcus aureus. Clin Infect Dis. 2011;53(4):334–40.

94. Bradbury T, Fehring TK, Taunton M, Hanssen A, Azzam K, Parvizi J, Odum SM. The fate of acute methicillin-resistant Staphylococcus aureus periprosthetic knee infections treated by open debridement and retention of components. J Arthroplast. 2009;24(6 Suppl):101–4.

95. Fehring TK, Odum SM, Berend KR, Jiranek WA, Parvizi J, Bozic KJ, et al. Failure of irrigation and débridement for early postoperative periprosthetic infection. Clin Orthop Relat Res. 2013;471(1):250–7.

96. McPherson EJ, Woodson C, Holtom P, Roidis N, Shufelt C, Patzakis M. Periprosthetic total hip infection: outcomes using a staging system. Clin Orthop Relat Res. 2002;403:8–15.

97. Kubista B, Hartzler RU, Wood CM, Osmon DR, Hanssen AD, Lewallen DG. Reinfection after two-stage revision for periprosthetic infection of total knee arthroplasty. Int Orthop. 2012;36(1):65–71.

98. Benito N, Franco M, Ribera A, Soriano A, Rodriguez-Pardo D, Sorlí L, REIPI (Spanish Network for Research in Infectious Disease) Group for the Study of Prosthetic Joint Infections, et al. Time trends in the aetiology of prosthetic joint infections: a multicentre cohort study. Clin Microbiol Infect. 2016;22(8):732.e1–8.

99. Lora-Tamayo J, Murillo O, Iribarren JA, Soriano A, Sánchez-Somolinos M, Baraia-Etxaburu JM, REIPI Group for the Study of Prosthetic Infection, et al. A large multicenter study of methicillin-susceptible and methicillin-resistant Staphylococcus aureus prosthetic joint infections managed with implant retention. Clin Infect Dis. 2013;56(2):182–94.

100. Tornero E, Senneville E, Euba G, Petersdorf S, Rodriguez-Pardo D, Lakatos B, European Society Group of Infections on Artificial Implants (ESGIAI), et al. Characteristics of prosthetic joint infections due to Enterococcus sp. and predictors of failure: a multi-national study. Clin Microbiol Infect. 2014;20(11):1219–24.

101. Li G, Guo F, Ou Y, Dong G, Zhou W. Epidemiology and outcomes of surgical site infections following orthopedic surgery. Am J Infect Control. 2013;41(12):1268–71.

102. Benito N, Franco M, Coll P, Gálvez ML, Jordán M, López-Contreras J, et al. Etiology of surgical site infections after primary total joint arthroplasties. J Orthop Res. 2014;32(5):633–7.

103. Peel TN, Cheng AC, Buising KL, Choong PF. Microbiological aetiology, epidemiology, and clinical profile of prosthetic joint

infections: are current antibiotic prophylaxis guidelines effective? Antimicrob Agents Chemother. 2012;56(5):2386–91.

104. Berríos-Torres SI, Yi SH, Bratzler DW, Ma A, Mu Y, Zhu L, Jernigan JA. Activity of commonly used antimicrobial prophylaxis regimens against pathogens causing coronary artery bypass graft and arthroplasty surgical site infections in the United States, 2006–2009. Infect Control Hosp Epidemiol. 2014;35(3):231–9.

105. Lamagni T, Elgohari S, Harrington P. Trends in surgical site infections following orthopaedic surgery. Curr Opin Infect Dis. 2015;28(2):125–32.

106. European Centre for Disease Prevention and Control. Annual epidemiological report 2014. Antimicrobial resistance and healthcare-associated infections. Stockholm: ECDC. 2015.

107. Aggarwal VK, Bakhshi H, Ecker NU, Parvizi J, Gehrke T, Kendoff D. Organism profile in periprosthetic joint infection: pathogens differ at two arthroplasty infection referral centers in Europe and in the United States. J Knee Surg. 2014;27(5):399–406.

108. Rodríguez-Pardo D, Pigrau C, Lora-Tamayo J, Soriano A, del Toro MD, Cobo J, REIPI Group for the Study of Prosthetic Infection, et al. Gram-negative prosthetic joint infection: outcome of a debridement, antibiotics and implant retention approach. A large multicentre study. Clin Microbiol Infect. 2014;20(11):O911–9.

109. Benito N, Franco M, Ribera A, Soriana A, Pigrau C, Sorli L, REIPI Group for the Study of Prosthetic Joint Infection, et al. Aetiology of prosthetic joint infections (PJIs) according to the type of infection in a large multicenter cohort: impact of antimicrobial resistance (abstract EP099). 25th European congress of clinical microbiology and infectious diseases. Copenhagen, Denmark, 25–28 April 2015.

110. Parvizi J, Erkocak OF, Della Valle CJ. Culture-negative periprosthetic joint infection. J Bone Joint Surg Am. 2014;96(5):430–6.

111. Lora-Tamayo J, Euba G, Ribera A, Murillo O, Pedrero S, García-Somoza D, et al. Infected hip hemiarthroplasties and total hip arthroplasties: differential findings and prognosis. J Infect. 2013;67(6):536–44.

112. Benito N, Mur I, Ribera A, Soriano D, Rodriguez-Pardo D, Sorli G, et al. Microbial aetiology of hip hemiarthroplasty (HHA) infections versus those associated with total hip arthroplasty (THA): impact of antimicrobial resistance (abstract

P0507). 26th European congress of clinical microbiology and infectious diseases. Amsterdam, Netherlands, 9–12 April 2016.

113. del Toro MD, Nieto I, Guerrero F, Corzo J, del Arco A, Palomino J, et al. Are hip hemiarthroplasty and total hip arthroplasty infections different entities? The importance of hip fractures. Eur J Clin Microbiol Infect Dis. 2014;33(8):1439–48.

114. Gristina AG. Biomaterial-centered infection: microbial adhesion versus tissue integration. Science. 1987;237(4822):1588–95.

115. Costerton JW. Biofilm theory can guide the treatment of device-related orthopaedic infections. Clin Orthop Relat Res. 2005;437:7–11.

116. Esteban J, Cordero-Ampuero J. Treatment of prosthetic osteoarticular infections. Expert Opin Pharmacother. 2011;12(6):899–912.

117. Katsikogianni M, Missirlis YF. Concise review of mechanisms of bacterial adhesion to biomaterials and of techniques used in estimating bacteria-material interactions. Eur Cell Mater. 2004;8:37–57.

118. Darouiche RO. Device-associated infections: a macro-problem that starts with microadherence. Clin Infect Dis. 2001;33(9):1567–72.

119. Esteban J, Pérrez-Tanoira R, Pérez-Jorge C, Gémez-Barrena E. Bacterial adherence to biomaterials used in surgical procedures. In: Kon K, Rai M, editors. Microbiology for surgical infections: diagnosis, prognosis, and treatment. London: Academic/Elsevier; 2014. p. 41–60.

120. Arciola CR, Visai L, Testoni F, Arciola S, Campoccia D, Speziale P, Montanaro L. Concise survey of Staphylococcus aureus virulence factors that promote adhesion and damage to peri-implant tissues. Int J Artif Organs. 2011;34(9):771–80.

121. Rohde H, Burandt EC, Siemssen N, Frommelt L, Burdelski C, Wurster S, et al. Polysaccharide intercellular adhesin or protein factors in biofilm accumulation of Staphylococcus epidermidis and Staphylococcus aureus isolated from prosthetic hip and knee joint infections. Biomaterials. 2007;28(9):1711–20.

122. Campoccia D, Montanaro L, Arciola CR. A review of the biomaterials technologies for infection-resistant surfaces. Biomaterials. 2013;34(34):8533–54.

123. Costerton JW, Montanaro L, Arciola CR. Biofilm in implant infections: its production and regulation. Int J Artif Organs. 2005;28(11):1062–8.

124. Flemming H-C, Wingender J, Szewzyk U, Steinberg P, Rice SA, Kjelleberg S. Biofilms: an emergent form of bacterial life. Nat Rev Microbiol. 2016;14(9):563–75.

125. Perez-Jorge C, Gomez-Barrena E, Horcajada J-P, Puig-Verdie L, Esteban J. Drug treatments for prosthetic joint infections in the era of multidrug resistance. Expert Opin Pharmacother. 2016;17(9):1233–46.

126. Molina-Manso D, del Prado G, Ortiz-Pérez A, Manrubia-Cobo M, Gómez-Barrena E, Cordero-Ampuero J, Esteban J. In vitro susceptibility to antibiotics of staphylococci in biofilms isolated from orthopaedic infections. Int J Antimicrob Agents. 2013;41(6):521–3.

127. Drancourt M, Stein A, Argenson JN, Zannier A, Curvale G, Raoult D. Oral rifampin plus ofloxacin for treatment of Staphylococcus-infected orthopedic implants. Antimicrob Agents Chemother. 1993;37(6):1214–8.

128. Broekhuizen CA, Sta M, Vandenbroucke-Grauls CM, Zaat SA. Microscopic detection of viable Staphylococcus epidermidis in peri-implant tissue in experimental biomaterial-associated infection, identified by bromodeoxyuridine incorporation. Infect Immun. 2010;78(3):954–62.

129. Tande AJ, Osmon DR, Greenwood-Quaintance KE, Mabry TM, Hanssen AD, Patel R. Clinical characteristics and outcomes of prosthetic joint infection caused by small colony variant staphylococci. MBio. 2014;5(5):e01910–4.

130. Proctor RA, von Eiff C, Kahl BC, Becker K, McNamara P, Herrmann M, Peters G. Small colony variants: a pathogenic form of bacteria that facilitates persistent and recurrent infections. Nat Rev Microbiol. 2006;4(4):295–305.

Chapter 3
Prosthetic Joint Infection: Diagnosis Update

Trisha Peel and Robin Patel

3.1 Background

It is well recognised that the diagnosis of prosthetic joint infections (PJIs) remains a challenging aspect of management for these infections. This is due to a number of interrelated issues: the lack of a perfect diagnostic reference standard, the presence of biofilm (which impedes both diagnostic and treatment strategies), challenges differentiating pathogens from contaminants, the overlap in symptomatology of septic and aseptic failure and the particular challenges for diagnosis of shoulder arthroplasty infections due to the prevalence of *Cutibacterium acnes* (previously known as *Propionibacterium acnes*) in this specific setting.

T. Peel (✉)
Department of Infectious Diseases, Monash University
and Alfred Health, Melbourne, Victoria, Australia
e-mail: trisha.peel@monash.edu

R. Patel
Divisions of Clinical Microbiology and Infectious Diseases,
Departments of Laboratory Medicine & Pathology and Medicine,
Mayo Clinic, Rochester, MN, USA

© Springer International Publishing AG 2018
T. Peel (ed.), *Prosthetic Joint Infections*,
https://doi.org/10.1007/978-3-319-65250-4_3

In recent years, the Musculoskeletal Infection Society (MSIS) and the Infectious Diseases Society of America (IDSA) have published criteria for the diagnosis of PJI [1, 2]. These criteria are an important development to allow a more unified approach in the diagnosis of infection. The MSIS diagnosis was refined further following the International Consensus Meeting on Periprosthetic Joint Infections [3]. Comparison of the three criteria is outlined in Table 3.1. The major difference between the IDSA and the MSIS criteria is the diagnostic weight of intraoperative purulence and

TABLE 3.1 Prosthetic joint infection diagnosis according to the Infectious Diseases Society of America (IDSA) criteria (Osmon et al. [1]), the original Musculoskeletal Infection Society (MSIS) criteria [2] and the revised MSIS criteria (Parvizi and Gehrke [3])

IDSA criteria

One or more of the following are present:

1. Indistinguishable microorganism isolated from two or more periprosthetic fluid or tissue samples

AND/OR

2. Sinus tract communicating with the affected joint

AND/OR

3. Intraoperative purulence

AND/OR

4. Acute inflammation on histologic examination

Original MSIS criteria

One or more of the following are present:

1. Indistinguishable microorganism isolated from two or more periprosthetic fluid or tissue samples

AND/OR

2. Sinus tract communicating with affected joint or

AND/OR

TABLE 3.1 (continued)

3. *Four of the following are present*:

   (a) Elevated serum C-reactive protein (CRP) and erythrocyte sedimentation rate (ESR)

   (b) Elevated synovial fluid leucocyte count

   (c) Elevated synovial fluid polymorphonuclear leucocyte percentage

   (d) Intraoperative purulence

   (e) Greater than five neutrophils per high-power field in 5 high-power fields observed from histologic analysis of periprosthetic tissue at 400× magnification

   (f) Isolation of a microorganism from a single periprosthetic fluid or tissue specimen

Revised MSIS criteria

One or more of the following are present:

1. Indistinguishable microorganism isolated on two or more periprosthetic fluid or tissue samples

AND/OR

2. Sinus tract communicating with affected joint

AND/OR

Three of the following are present:

   1. Elevated serum CRP and ESR

   2. Elevated synovial fluid leucocyte count or ++ change on leucocyte esterase test strip

   3. Elevated synovial fluid polymorphonuclear leucocyte percentage

   4. Greater than five neutrophils per high-power field in 5 high-power fields observed from histologic analysis of periprosthetic tissue at 400× magnification

   5. Single positive culture

histopathology findings, considered major criteria using the IDSA scheme compared to minor criteria using the MSIS scheme [1–3]. According to the revised MSIS criteria, the presence of intraoperative purulence is no longer considered a criterion for PJI [3]. In the justification provided by the International Consensus Meeting, intraoperative purulence was viewed as too subjective and non-specific [4]. In particular, turbid fluids may be observed intraoperatively with other conditions, most notably with metallosis [4, 5]. This is supported by a study by Alijanipour et al. in which the presence of purulence had a sensitivity of 82% but a low specificity of 32% [5].

The revised MSIS criteria also attempted to provide clarity for the cut-offs for different biochemical markers, according to the acuity of the infection, as outlined in Table 3.2 [3]. The thresholds described in the revised MSIS criteria will be discussed in more detail in this chapter. Finally, authors of all three criteria clearly state that, in patients not meeting diagnostic criteria, PJI may still be present and therefore clinical judgement is advocated [1–4].

TABLE 3.2 Diagnostic thresholds for minor criteria according to the revised musculoskeletal infection society definition (Adapted from Parvizi and Gehrke [3])

Criterion	Acute prosthetic joint infection (<90 days)	Chronic prosthetic joint infection (>90 days)
Erythrocyte sedimentation rate (ESR) (mm/h)	No threshold determined	30
C-reactive protein (CRP) (mg/L)	100	10
Synovial leucocyte count (cells/µL)	10,000	3000
Synovial polymorphonuclear leucocyte percent	90	80

Another challenge with diagnosis of PJI is the crossover between pathogen and contaminant. Coagulase-negative staphylococci, such as *Staphylococcus epidermidis*, are the most common causes of PJI. Conversely coagulase-negative staphylococci are the major cause of contamination of microbiological specimens. For example, in a large cohort study with 369 subjects undertaken at Mayo Clinic, Rochester, MN, USA, 25% of infections were due to coagulase-negative *Staphylococcus* species, isolated in 29 of the 117 subjects meeting the IDSA criteria for infection. However, coagulase-negative *Staphylococcus* species were the most common contaminants, isolated in 33 of the 252 subjects (13%) of patients not meeting the IDSA criteria for PJI [6]. Diagnostic tests that clearly differentiate whether an isolated microorganism is a true pathogen or a contaminant do not exist in clinical practice; therefore, it frequently falls to clinical judgement to assess the significance of isolated organisms.

Further compounding PJI diagnosis is the overlap in symptomatology between septic failure (i.e. PJI) and aseptic failure; in particular, pain is the most common symptom of PJI and, however, is also the predominant symptom of aseptic failure [7, 8]. The challenge in differentiating between aseptic and septic failure based on clinical history and examination alone results in a need for diagnostic testing [7].

Finally, the diagnosis of shoulder arthroplasty infections is particularly challenging. *C. acnes* is the predominant organism associated with shoulder PJI [9]. This organism behaves differently compared to other organisms, such as *Staphylococcus aureus*. It causes more indolent infections and does not incite the same inflammatory reaction as other organisms, and isolation of some strains may require extended incubation of microbiological cultures, a situation that is, in part, method dependent [10–12].

In the last decade, there has been an upsurge of studies examining optimisation of PJI diagnosis, with significant advances having been made in PJI diagnosis and interpretation of results of diagnostic testing. This chapter will review the current state of PJI diagnosis.

3.2   Clinical Diagnosis

3.2.1   Diagnostic Criteria

As noted by the authors of the PJI diagnostic criteria, clinical assessment and judgement remain of critical importance for the diagnosis of these infections. Two main classifications systems have been developed to assist in the assessment of patients. Zimmerli et al. classified PJI as "early" developing in the first 3 months after surgery, "delayed" occurring 3 to 24 months after surgery and "late" occurring greater than 24 months after joint replacement surgery [7]. A similar classification system was developed by Tsukayama et al., with PJI classified as "early postoperative" developing within 4 weeks of the index procedure, "late chronic" developing after 4 weeks of the index procedure with an insidious clinical presentation and "acute haematogenous" developing after 4 weeks of the index procedure with an acute onset of symptoms [13]. These classification systems loosely relate to symptomatology and likely pathogens associated with PJI and inform management strategies, particularly with the classification system developed by Tsukayama and colleagues (Table 3.3) [3, 13].

3.2.2   Clinical Presentation

In early infections, patients typically present with surgical wound complications, such as purulent discharge, erythema and swelling of the affected joint [7, 14–16]. Early infections are typically associated with organisms such as *S. aureus* [7, 14–16]. In acute haematogenous infections, patients often report sudden onset of pain at the site of a prosthetic joint that has been previously asymptomatic, with or without swelling or fever [7, 14–16]. Organisms such as *Streptococcus* species and *S. aureus* are classic organisms associated with acute haematogenous PJIs [7, 14–16]. In late chronic infections, many of the typical symptoms of infection are absent. Pain is the predominant feature, with patients reporting a history of slowly increasing pain involving the prosthetic joint [7, 14–16]. A discharging sinus, when present, is typically associated with chronic, indolent presentations [2, 7,

TABLE 3.3 Typical clinical features, biomarker profile and microorganisms according to prosthetic joint infection classification proposed by Tsukayama et al. [13] and the revised MSIS criteria (Parvizi and Gehrke [3])

Classification	Days from surgery (days)	Clinical features	Serum CRP (mg/L)	Serum ESR	Synovial leukocyte count	Synovial PMN%	Typical pathogens
Early postoperative	≤30	• Purulent discharge/ ooze	>100	Nil threshold determined	>10,000 cells/ μL	>90	Staphylococcus aureus
		• Erythema					
		• Swelling of index joint					
		• Dehiscence					Gram-negative bacilli
		• Pain					
		• ±Fever					
Late chronic	≥30	• Insidious onset of pain ("grumblers")	>10	>30 mm/h	>3000 cells/ μL	>80	Coagulase-negative staphylococci
		• ±Sinus tract					Cutibacterium acnes

(continued)

TABLE 3.3 (continued)

Classification	Days from surgery (days)	Clinical features	Serum CRP (mg/L)	Serum ESR	Synovial leukocyte count	Synovial PMN%	Typical pathogens
Acute haematogenous	≥30	• Sudden onset of pain • Swelling of index joint • ±Fever	>100	Nil threshold determined	>10,000 cells/ μL	>90	Staphylococcus aureus Streptococcus species

CRP C-reactive protein, *ESR* erythrocyte sedimentation rate, *PMN* polymorphonuclear leukocytes

13, 15]. These infections are classically associated with coagulase-negative staphylococci [16]. As previously discussed, *C. acnes* has a predilection for infecting shoulder joints and tends to cause indolent infections [17–20]. Classic features of infection are frequently absent, with pain and stiffness of the shoulder joint being the predominant symptoms. Bruising along the surgical wound has been described as a pathognomonic sign of *C. acnes* shoulder arthroplasty infection [17–20].

Regardless of which classification system is applied, classification of PJI influences management decisions; debridement and retention of the prosthesis is a potential treatment option for early and acute haematogenous infections but not for delayed or late chronic infections [1, 4, 7].

The timing of prosthesis failure also aids clinical acumen. In a prospective cohort study by Portillo and colleagues, the underlying indication for prosthesis revision was examined, comparing the median time for revision due to PJI, mechanical failure (such as dislocation) and aseptic failure. Overall, the need for revision within 2 years of the index procedure was highly predictive of PJI with a calculated risk ratio of 2.9 (95% confidence interval 1.8–4.8). The authors also noted that infections occurring after 2 years were more likely to be acute haematogenous infections and were easily clinically distinguishable from aseptic failure [21].

3.3   Blood Inflammatory Markers

3.3.1   Blood White Cell Count

A number of studies have assessed the utility of blood markers in the diagnosis of PJI. Elevated blood white cell count is a poor predictor of infection; in most series, fewer than 10% of patients with PJI have an elevated peripheral blood white cell count [7, 8, 22]. In a systematic review and meta-analysis performed by Berbari and colleagues, the pooled sensitivity of an elevated peripheral blood white cell count was 45% (95% confidence interval 41–49%) [22]. Two studies published subsequent to the meta-analysis by Berbari et al. have demonstrated diverse results (Table 3.4) [1, 2, 12, 22–30]. Glehr and

TABLE 3.4 Selected literature review of test performance for serum white cell count, C-reactive protein and erythrocyte sedimentation rate

Biomarker	Reference	Joint(s)	Chronicity[a]	Number[b]	Threshold[c]	Prosthetic joint infection criteria	Sensitivity (%)	Specificity (%)
White cell count (WCC)								
	Berbari et al. [22][d]	Knee and hip	Not specified	3909	Not specified	Not specified	45	87
	Glehr et al. [23]	Knee and hip	Not specified	124	WCC > 7355 cells/μL	Original MSIS criteria [2]	73	72
	Randau et al. [24]	Knee and hip	Not specified	120	WCC > 10,300 cells/μL	IDSA criteria [1]	21	94
C-reactive protein (CRP)								
	Berbari et al. [22][d]	Knee and hip	Not specified	3909	Not specified	Not specified	88	74
	Glehr et al. [23]	Knee and hip	Not specified	124	Not specified	Original MSIS criteria [2]	84	79
	Randau et al. [24]	Knee and hip	Not specified	120	CRP >9.1 mg/L	Osmon et al. [1] IDSA criteria	62	83
	Ettinger et al. [25]	Knee, hip and shoulder	Chronic (>4 weeks)	98	CRP >0.3 mg/dL	Original MSIS criteria [2]	80	64

Study	Joint	Acute/Chronic	N	CRP	Reference standard	Sensitivity	Specificity
Alijanipour et al. [26]	Knee and hip	Acute (<4 weeks)	1773	CRP >23.5 mg/L	Original MSIS criteria [2]	87	94
Bedair et al. [27]	Knee	Acute (<6 weeks)	146	CRP ≥166 mg/dL	*One or more of the following:* 1. Intraoperative purulence 2. Positive culture on solid media	53	86
Alijanipour et al. [26]	Knee	Chronic (>4 weeks)	759	CRP >23.5 mg/L	Original MSIS criteria [2]	92	94
Piper et al. [12]	Knee	Not specified	297	CRP >14.5 mg/L	*One or more of the following:* 1. Intraoperative purulence 2. Histology consistent with infection 3. Sinus tract 4. Positive tissue *and* sonicate culture	79	88

(continued)

TABLE 3.4 (continued)

Biomarker	Reference	Joint(s)	Chronicity[a]	Number[b]	Threshold[c]	Prosthetic joint infection criteria	Sensitivity (%)	Specificity (%)
	Yi et al. [28]	Hip	Acute (<6 weeks)	73	CRP > 93 mg/L	*One or more of the following:* 1. Organism isolated from ≥2 cultures 2. Sinus tract 3. *Two of the following:* (a) Intraoperative purulence (b) Histology consistent with infection (c) Single culture positive	88	100
	Alijanipour et al. [26]	Hip	Chronic (>4 weeks)	1203	CRP >13.5 mg/L	Original MSIS criteria [2]	90	88

Piper et al. [12]	Hip	Not specified	221	CRP >10.3 mg/L	One or more of the following: 1. Intraoperative purulence 2. Histology consistent with infection 3. Sinus tract 4. Positive tissue and sonicate culture	74	79
Piper et al. [12]	Shoulder	Not specified	64	CRP >7 mg/L	One or more of the following: 1. Intraoperative purulence 2. Histology consistent with infection 3. Sinus tract 4. Positive tissue and sonicate culture	63	73
Erythrocyte sedimentation rate (ESR)							
Berbari et al. [22][d]	Knee and hip	Not specified	3909	Not specified	Not specified	75	70

(continued)

Table 3.4 (continued)

Biomarker	Reference	Joint(s)	Chronicity[a]	Number[b]	Threshold[c]	Prosthetic joint infection criteria	Sensitivity (%)	Specificity (%)
	Alijanipour et al. [26]	Knee and hip	Acute (<4 weeks)	1773	ESR >54.5 mm/h	Original MSIS criteria [2]	80	93
	Bedair et al. [27]	Knee	Acute (<6 weeks)	146	ESR ≥120 mm/h	*One or more of the following:* 1. Intraoperative purulence 2. Positive culture on solid media	16	94
	Alijanipour et al. [26]	Knee	Chronic (>4 weeks)	759	ESR >46.5 mm/h	Original MSIS criteria [2]	87	87
	Piper et al. [12]	Knee	Not specified	297	ESR >19 mm/h	*One or more of the following:* 1. Intraoperative purulence 2. Histology consistent with infection 3. Sinus tract 4. Positive tissue *and* sonicate culture	89	74

Yi et al. [28]	Hip	Acute (< 6 weeks)	73	ESR > 44 mm/h	*One or more of the following:* 1. Organism isolated from ≥2 cultures 2. Sinus tract 3. *Two of the following:* (a) Intraoperative purulence (b) Histology consistent with infection (c) Single culture positive	92	53
Alijanipour et al. [26]	Hip	Chronic (>4 weeks)	1203	ESR >48.5 mm/h	Original MSIS criteria [2]	78	90

(continued)

TABLE 3.4 (continued)

Biomarker	Reference	Joint(s)	Chronicity[a]	Number[b]	Threshold[c]	Prosthetic joint infection criteria	Sensitivity (%)	Specificity (%)
	Piper et al. [12]	Hip	Not specified	221	ESR >13 mm/h	*One or more of the following;* 1. Intraoperative purulence 2. Histology consistent with infection 3. Sinus tract 4. Positive tissue *and* sonicate culture	82	60
	Piper et al. [12]	Shoulder	Not specified	64	ESR >26 mm/h	*One or more of the following:* 1. Intraoperative purulence 2. Histology consistent with infection 3. Sinus tract 4. Positive tissue *and* sonicate culture	32	93

Combined CRP and ESR

	Joint	Acute/chronic	N	Threshold	Reference standard	Sens	Spec
Austin et al. [29]	Knee	Not specified	296	CRP >10 mg/L *and* ESR >30 mm/h	*One or more of the following:* 1. Positive intraoperative cultures 2. Synovial white cell count >1760 cells/μL *and* PMN% >73% 3. Sinus tract	96	56
Piper et al. [12]	Knee	Not specified	297	CRP >14.5 mg/L *or* ESR > 19 mm/h	*One or more of the following:* 1. Intraoperative purulence 2. Histology consistent with infection 3. Sinus tract 4. Positive tissue *and* sonicate culture	94	69
Aljanipour et al. [26]	Knee	Acute and chronic	759	CRP >23.5 mg/L *and* ESR >46.5 mm/h	Original MSIS criteria [2]	89	85

(continued)

TABLE 3.4 (continued)

Biomarker	Reference	Joint(s)	Chronicity[a]	Number[b]	Threshold[c]	Prosthetic joint infection criteria	Sensitivity (%)	Specificity (%)
	Alijanipour et al. [26]	Hip	Acute and chronic	1203	CRP >13.5 mg/L *and* ESR >48.5 mm/h	Original MSIS criteria [2]	75	84
	Schinsky et al. [30]	Hip	Acute and chronic	235	ESR >30 mm/h *and* CRP >10 mg/dL	*Two of the following three:* 1. Positive intraoperative culture 2. Gross purulence 3. Histology consistent with infection	90	91
	Piper et al. [12]	Hip	Not specified	221	CRP > 10.3 mg/L *or* ESR > 13 mm/h	*One or more of the following:* 1. Intraoperative purulence 2. Histology consistent with infection 3. Sinus tract 4. Positive tissue *and* sonicate culture	88	55

| Piper et al. [12] | Shoulder | Not specified | 64 | CRP > 7 mg/L or ESR > 26 mm/h | *One or more of the following:* 1. Intraoperative purulence 2. Histology consistent with infection 3. Sinus tract 4. Positive tissue *and* sonicate culture | 63 | 73 |

[a]Unless otherwise specified, chronicity refers to the time from index prosthetic joint surgery until prosthetic joint revision surgery

[b]Number of revision arthroplasties

[c]Threshold based on ROC analysis when provided

[d]Meta-analysis

MSIS Musculoskeletal Infection Society, *IDSA* Infectious Diseases Society of America colleagues examined blood markers in patients undergoing hip or knee revision surgery [23]. The study included 124 revision arthroplasties, of which 78 met the original MSIS diagnostic criteria for PJI. Applying a cut-off of 7355 white cells/µL, the sensitivity was 73%, higher than the sensitivity reported in the meta-analysis. In contrast, in a second study by Randau and colleagues, applying a threshold of 10,300 cell/µL, the sensitivity of peripheral blood white cell count was only 21.3% (95% confidence interval 10.7–35.7%) [24]. Despite the low sensitivity, measurement of blood white cell count is commonly performed as part of standard preoperative workup.

3.3.2 C-Reactive Protein and Erythrocyte Sedimentation Rate

Other biochemical tests, such as erythrocyte sedimentation rate (ESR) and serum C-reactive protein (CRP), are more useful diagnostic investigations for PJI [1–4, 22]. These tests are inexpensive, widely available and commonly performed in this clinical setting; furthermore, clinicians are familiar with their interpretation [31]. In the study by Berbari et al., the pooled sensitivity of ESR was 75% (95% confidence interval 72–77%), and serum CRP was 88% (95% confidence interval 86–90%) for the detection of lower limb PJI [22]. In addition, studies have examined the sensitivity of combining ESR and serum CRP. In a study by Schinsky et al. examining 235 revision total hip arthroplasties, the combination of elevated ESR and serum CRP had a sensitivity of 90% and specificity of 91% [30]. Similarly, Austin et al. examined blood markers in 296 patients undergoing revision total knee arthroplasty; combining ESR and serum CRP had a sensitivity of 96%; however, the specificity was much lower at 56% [29]. As noted by Berbari et al., the cut-off values for these inflammatory markers differed in studies [22]. In addition, the thresholds for these markers differ between early and late chronic infections and by prosthesis location [26].

In attempt to provide clarity, the recent International Consensus Meeting specified cut-offs, distinguishing between acute PJI (defined as less than 90 days) and chronic PJI (defined as greater than 90 days). For CRP, the threshold for acute infections was 100 mg/L and 10 mg/L for chronic infections. For ESR, the threshold for chronic infections was 30 mm/h: no threshold was stipulated for acute infections, due to poor specificity of ESR in the early postoperative period [3, 4]. There is a paucity of data to support the thresholds suggested, and the data that does exist is conflicting. In the study by Alijanipour et al. examining 1962 patients undergoing total hip or knee revision arthroplasties, 273 of whom underwent revision for PJI, the inflammatory markers differed between early and late chronic infections with higher values noted in early infections [26]. In addition, the median CRP was higher in knee PJI (133, interquartile range [IQR] 40–207) compared to hip PJI (84, IQR 55–101; $P < 0.0001$). For late chronic knee infections, the optimal cut-off values based on receiver operating characteristic (ROC) analysis for CRP was 23.5 mg/L with a sensitivity of 92% and specificity of 94% and for ESR 46.5 mm/h (sensitivity 87% and specificity 87%) [26]. In late chronic hip infections, Alijanipour and colleagues suggested a cut-off of 13.5 mg/L for CRP (sensitivity 90% and specificity 88%); however, the threshold suggested for ESR (48.5 mm/h) was associated with reduced sensitivity—78% [26]. For early infections, Alijanipour et al. suggested a threshold of 54.5 mm/h for ESR (sensitivity 80% and specificity of 93%) and 23.5 mg/L for CRP (sensitivity 87% and specificity 94%) for both hips and knee joints [26].

In contrast, studies by Bedair et al. suggested an optimal CRP threshold of 166 mg/L for early postoperative knee infections (sensitivity of 53%, 95% confidence interval 43–62%, and specificity 86%, 95% confidence interval 79–92%). The ESR threshold of 120 mm/h was associated with a sensitivity of 16% (95% confidence interval 9–23%) and specificity of 94%, (95% confidence interval 90–99%) [27].

In patients undergoing hip revision surgery for early postoperative infections, Yi et al. suggested optimal cut-offs for

CRP of 93 mg/L for hips (sensitivity 88%, 95% confidence interval 77–98%) [28]. Similar to the observations of Bedair et al., the optimal cut-off for ESR was 44 mm/h with excellent sensitivity (92%, 95% confidence interval 83–100%) but low specificity (53%, 95% confidence interval 38–69%) [28]. The observed poor specificity with ESR in acute infections may relate to the fact that ESR is elevated in the postoperative period in uncomplicated joint surgery. Indeed, in an early study by Shih et al., ESR remained elevated out to a year in a small subset of patients [32]. In contrast, CRP peaks on day 2 and returns to normal within 3 weeks [31–34]. In addition, there may be potential overlap with other conditions that elevate inflammatory markers, such as rheumatoid arthritis [22]. Yi and colleagues also observed that combining ESR and CRP did not improve test performance in the acute setting [28]. Of further interest, in a study by Bracken et al., which compared CRP and ESR in 44 patients with fungal PJI compared to 59 patients with bacterial PJI, it was noted that these inflammatory markers did not differ between fungal and bacterial PJI [35].

These measures are of limited clinical benefit in predicting shoulder arthroplasty infections; in a study by Piper et al., applying a cut-off of 26 mm/h for ESR and 7 mg/L for CRP, these markers had a sensitivity of 32% for ESR and 63% for CRP and a specificity of 93% for ESR and 73% for CRP [12]. In 23% of shoulder infections, the ESR and CRP were not elevated [12]. Similarly, in a study by Topolski et al., ESR (applying a cut-off of 22 mm/h) and CRP (applying a cut-off of 1 dL/L) were only elevated in 14% and 25% of patients, respectively [36].

The spectrum of reported test performance of these serum biomarkers is outlined in Table 3.4. In addition, Table 3.4 also highlights the range of definitions applied for PJI, thereby hampering the direct comparison of results between studies. Notwithstanding, ESR and CRP are relatively useful tests, given their broad availability and reasonable sensitivity; however, the optimal cut-offs according to chronicity of infection and location of the index prosthetic joint still require further

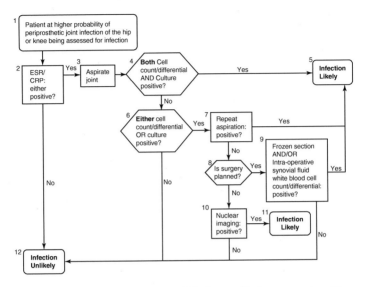

FIGURE 3.1 American Academy of Orthopaedic Surgeons algorithm for patients with higher probability of hip or knee periprosthetic joint infection (From AAOS [37], with permission)

study. In addition, the specificity of ESR is poor, particularly in early postoperative infections. As previously discussed, elevated ESR and CRP are minor criteria for the MSIS and revised MSIS diagnostic criteria [2, 3]. Of interest, in the diagnostic algorithm proposed by the American Academy of Orthopaedic Surgeons (Fig. 3.1), CRP and ESR are suggested as initial tests to exclude the diagnosis of PJI; however, given the variation in reported sensitivity, specificity and predictive value of these tests, the validity of this is unclear [37].

3.3.3 Interleukin-6, Procalcitonin C and Tumour Necrosis Factor-α

Other studied serum biochemical markers of infection include interleukin-6, tumour necrosis factor-α (TNF-α) and procalcitonin C (Table 3.5) [1, 2, 22–25, 38, 39].

TABLE 3.5 Selected literature review of test performance for serum interleukin-6, procalcitonin and tumour necrosis factor-α

Biomarker Reference	Joint(s)	Chronicity[a]	Number[b]	Threshold[c]	Prosthetic joint infection criteria	Sensitivity (%)	Specificity (%)
Interleukin-6 (IL-6)							
Berbari et al. [22][d]	Knee and hip	Not specified	3909	Not specified	Not specified	97	91
Glehr et al. [23]	Knee and hip	Not specified	124	IL-6 > 4.7 pg/mL	Original MSIS criteria [2]	81	68
Ettinger et al. [25]	Knee, hip and shoulder	Chronic (>4 weeks)	98	IL-6 > 5.12 pg/mL	Original MSIS criteria [2]	80	88
Randau et al. [24]	Knee and hip	Not specified	120	IL-6 > 2.6 pg/mL	Osmon et al. [1] IDSA criteria	79	58
Procalcitonin C (PCT)							
Glehr et al. [23]	Knee and hip	Not specified	124	PCT >0.75 ng/mL	Original MSIS criteria [2]	48	100
Bottner et al. [38]	Knee and hip	Acute and chronic	78	PCT >0.3 ng/mL	1. Positive intraoperative culture 2. Histology consistent with infection	33	98

Yuan et al. [39]	Hip	Not specified	74	PCT >0.5 ng/mL	Two of the following three: 1. Positive intraoperative culture 2. Intraoperative purulence 3. Histology consistent with infection	80	74
Ettinger et al. [25]	Knee, hip and shoulder	Chronic (>4 weeks)	98	PCT >0.025 ng/mL	Original MSIS criteria [2]	90	28
Randau et al. [24]	Knee and hip	Not specified	120	PCT > 46 ng/mL	Osmon et al. [1] IDSA criteria	13	100
Tumour necrosis factor-alpha (TNF-α)							
Bottner et al. [38]	Knee and hip	Acute and chronic	78	TNF-α >40.0 ng/mL	1. Positive intraoperative culture *and* 2. Histology consistent with infection	43	94

(continued)

TABLE 3.5 (continued)

Biomarker	Reference	Joint(s)	Chronicity[a]	Number[b]	Threshold[c]	Prosthetic joint infection criteria	Sensitivity (%)	Specificity (%)
	Ettinger et al. [25]	Knee, hip, and shoulder	Chronic (>4 weeks)	98	TNF-α >11.9 pg/mL	Original MSIS criteria [2]	35	86

[a]Unless otherwise specified, chronicity refers to the time from index prosthetic joint surgery until prosthetic joint revision surgery

[b]Number of revision arthroplasties

[c]Threshold based on ROC analysis when provided

[d]Meta-analysis

MSIS Musculoskeletal Infection Society

Interleukin-6 and TNF-α are cytokines released by mono-cytes and macrophages in the setting of infection [38]. Procalcitonin C is a precursor of calcitonin that has been shown to be a specific marker for a number of bacterial infections, including pneumonia and sepsis [40]. Bottner et al. compared the diagnostic utility of interleukin-6, TNF-α and procalcitonin C in 78 patients undergoing revision arthroplasties [38]. According to this study, patients were diagnosed with infection based on their having positive cultures or histological evidence of infection; however, details as to the exact aspects of these criteria were not further specified [38]. The authors noted that these serum biomarkers were all significantly elevated in patients meeting the above definition of infection, compared to patients with "aseptic loosening". The observed sensitivity and specificity of interleukin-6 were 95% and 87%, respectively [38]. Bottner et al. also noted that in six of the seven patients with false-positive interleukin-6 results, there was associated polyethylene wear and osteolysis, which may limit its utility [38].

Interleukin-6 is elevated in the postoperative period for primary arthroplasty; however, it returns to normal levels within 2 days of the operation [38]. Therefore, there is potential diagnostic utility of interleukin-6 over CRP and ESR in the early postoperative period if infection is suspected [41, 42]. In the meta-analysis by Berbari and colleagues, the pooled sensitivity and specificity for interleukin-6 was 97% (95% confidence interval 93–99%) with a pooled specificity of 91% (95% confidence interval 87–94%) [22]. In addition to the study by Bottner et al., the meta-analysis included two other small studies [22]. In a more recent study by Glehr et al. which was not included in the meta-analysis, preoperative performance of interleukin-6 did not predict infection [23]. Applying an optimal cut-off of 4.7 pg/mL, interleukin-6 had a sensitivity of 81% and specificity of 68%. Similar sensitivities have been reported in other studies [24, 25]. Interleukin-6 is not routinely available in most commercial laboratories, and the applicability and value of this marker remain unclear [31].

Five conflicting studies have examined procalcitonin in the setting of PJI; in the aforementioned study by Bottner et al., the sensitivity was 33% and specificity was 98% [38]. In contrast, in a study by Yuan et al. recruiting 71 patients undergoing revision hip arthroplasty, applying a cut-off of 0.5 ng/mL, the sensitivity of procalcitonin C was 80.0% and specificity was 73.9% [39]. As in the study by Bottner et al., the study by Glehr et al. demonstrated poor sensitivity of procalcitonin (48%); however, the specificity was 100% when a cut-off of 0.75 ng/mL was applied [23]. In the study by Randau and colleagues, procalcitonin performance was very poor (12.9%; 95% confidence interval 3.6–29.8%) when a higher threshold of 46 ng/mL was applied [40]. All studies noted no superiority of procalcitonin over CRP: Bottner et al. also noted that the cost of procalcitonin was 24 times higher than CRP [23, 38, 39]. Therefore, the value of procalcitonin in this clinical setting has not been established [24]. Finally Bottner et al. also examined the test characteristics of tumour necrosis factor-α, reporting a sensitivity of 43% and specificity of 94% applying a cut-off of 40.0 ng/mL [38]. These markers, interleukin-6, tumour necrosis factor-α and procalcitonin C, have not been incorporated into any diagnostic algorithm.

3.4   Synovial Fluid Characteristics

Synovial fluid characteristics can be used to assist in diagnosis of PJI (Table 3.6) [27, 28, 30, 43, 44]. The leucocyte composition in synovial fluid differs in patients with PJI compared to inflammatory conditions such as rheumatoid arthritis. In patients with PJI, there is a predominance of CD15-positive monocytes [45]. In comparison, T lymphocytes are the predominant cell type in inflammatory conditions [45].

TABLE 3.6 Selected literature review of test performance for synovial leukocyte count and polymorphonuclear leucocyte percentage

Biomarker	Reference	Joint(s)	Chronicity[a]	Number[b]	Threshold[c]	Prosthetic joint infection criteria	Sensitivity (%)	Specificity (%)
Synovial leucocyte count								
	Cipriano et al. [43]	Knee and hip	Chronic	871	>3450 cells/μL	Organism isolated from ≥2 cultures or *two of the following:* 1. Sinus tract 2. Intraoperative purulence 3. Histology consistent with infection	91	93
	Bedair et al. [27]	Knee	Acute (<6 weeks)	146	≥10,700 cells/μL	*One or more of the following:* 1. Intraoperative purulence 2. Positive culture on solid media	95	91

(continued)

TABLE 3.6 (continued)

Biomarker	Reference	Joint(s)	Chronicity[a]	Number[b]	Threshold[c]	Prosthetic joint infection criteria	Sensitivity (%)	Specificity (%)
	Trampuz et al. [44]	Knee	Chronic	133	>1700 cells/µL	*One or more of the following:* 1. Organism isolated from ≥2 cultures 2. Sinus tract 3. Purulence 4. Histology consistent with infection	94	88
	Yi et al. [28]	Hip	Acute (<6 weeks)	73	>12,800 cells/µL	*One or more of the following:* 1. Organism isolated from ≥2 cultures 2. Sinus tract 3. *Two of the following:* (a) Intraoperative purulence (b) Histology consistent with infection (c) Single culture positive	89	100

Polymorphonuclear leucocyte percentage

Study	Joint	Acute/chronic	Number	Threshold	Definition		
Schinsky et al. [30]	Hip	Acute and chronic	235	> 4200 cells/mL	*Two of the following three:* 1. Positive intraoperative culture 2. Gross purulence 3. Histology consistent with infection	84	93
Cipriano et al. [43]	Knee & hip	Chronic	871	>78%	1. Organism isolated from ≥2 cultures or 2. *Two of the following:* (a) Sinus tract (b) Intraoperative purulence (c) Histology consistent with infection	95.5	87
Bedair et al. [27]	Knee	Acute (<6 weeks)	146	>89%	*One or more of the following:* 1. Intraoperative purulence 2. Positive culture on solid media	84	69

(continued)

TABLE 3.6 (continued)

Biomarker	Reference	Joint(s)	Chronicity[a]	Number[b]	Threshold[c]	Prosthetic joint infection criteria	Sensitivity (%)	Specificity (%)
	Trampuz et al. [44]	Knee	Chronic	133	>65%	*One or more of the following:* 1. Organism isolated from ≥2 cultures 2. Sinus tract 3. Purulence 4. Histology 5. Consistent with infection	97	98
	Yi et al. [28]	Hip	Acute (<6 weeks)	73	>89%	*One or more of the following:* 1. Organism isolated from ≥2 cultures 2. Sinus tract 3. *Two of the following:* (a) Intraoperative purulence (b) Histology consistent with infection (c) Single culture positive	81	90

Schinsky et al. [30]	Hips	Acute and chronic	235	>80%	*Two of the following three:* 1. Positive intraoperative culture 2. Gross purulence 3. Histology consistent with infection	84	82

[a]Unless otherwise specified, chronicity refers to the time from index prosthetic joint surgery until prosthetic joint revision surgery

[b]Number of revision arthroplasties

[c]Threshold based on ROC analysis when provided

3.4.1 Synovial Leukocyte Count and Polymorphonuclear Percentage

As with inflammatory markers, the cellular profile of the synovial aspirate differs between early and chronic infections. In the acute setting, defined as infections occurring within 42 days of implantation, Yi et al. examined synovial aspirates in 73 patients undergoing total hip revision surgery within 6 weeks of surgery. Applying a modified version of the original MSIS criteria for infection (omitting inflammatory markers as a minor criterion), 36 patients met the diagnostic criteria for PJI [28]. In this study, the authors showed that a synovial leucocyte count of 12,800 cells/μL had a sensitivity of 89% (95% confidence interval 81–96%) and a specificity of 100% (95% confidence interval 100–100%) [28]. A polymorphonuclear leucocyte percentage of 89% had a sensitivity of 81% sensitivity (95% confidence interval 71–90%) and a specificity of 90% (83–97%) [28].

A further study by Bedair et al. involved 146 knee arthroplasty patients undergoing synovial aspiration within 6 weeks of surgery. Of note, Bedair et al. did not specify whether patients with inflammatory arthritis were excluded, which may impact the cellular profile [27]. In this study, patients were diagnosed with PJI if they had positive cultures or intraoperative purulence observed, with 19 patients meeting this definition of infection. Based on receiver-operator curve analysis, applying a threshold of 10,700 cells/μL, synovial leucocyte count had a sensitivity of 95% (95% confidence interval 91–98%) and specificity of 91% (95% confidence interval 87–96%) [27]. A threshold of 89% polymorphonuclear leucocytes had a sensitivity of 84% (95% confidence interval 78–90%); however, the specificity was lower (69%; 95% confidence interval 62–77%) [27].

Interpretation of these findings is challenging owing to the different PJI definitions applied and the lack of detail as to whether patients with inflammatory arthritis were specifically excluded. However, drawing on the results of these two studies, the revised MSIS criteria included synovial fluid characteristic as minor criteria, stipulating a cut-off for synovial leucocyte count of 10,000 cells/μL and polymorphonuclear percentage of 90% in acute infections. The new MSIS criteria however specify early infections as less than 90 days, which differs from the definitions applied by both Yi et al. and Bedair et al. [3, 27, 28]. Whether this alteration in timelines (i.e. 42 vs. 90 days) influences synovial fluid leucocyte count and polymorphonuclear leucocyte percentage is unknown.

In the setting of chronic infection, a number of studies have examined the optimal cut-off for synovial fluid leucocyte count and polymorphonuclear leucocyte percentage. An early study by Trampuz and colleagues examined the synovial fluid characteristics of 133 patients prior to total knee joint revision surgery [44]. In this study, patients with inflammatory arthritis were specifically excluded. The authors applied a definition for PJI that closely aligned with the subsequently published IDSA criteria, and overall, 34 patients in this cohort met this definition [1, 44]. Overall, a cut-off for synovial leucocyte count >1700 cells/μL had an excellent sensitivity (94%; 95% confidence interval 80–99%) and reasonable specificity (88%; 95% confidence interval 80–93%). A polymorphonuclear leucocyte percentage > 65% had a sensitivity of 97% (95% confidence interval 85–100%) and specificity of 98% (95% confidence interval 93–100%) [44]. In the corresponding revision hip arthroplasty cohort by Schinsky et al., involving 235 hip arthroplasties, a similar definition of PJI was applied, with the exception of exclusion of microbiological findings [30]. Fifty-five hips met this definition of infection. Applying a threshold of >4200 leucocyte count/mL, synovial fluid leucocyte count had a reported sensitivity of 84% (95% confidence interval 74–94%) and specificity of 93% (95% confidence interval 88–98%) [30]. Similarly a threshold of >80% synovial polymorphonuclear leukocytes had a sensitivity of 84% (95% confidence interval 74–93%) and specificity of 82% (95% confidence interval 76–89%) [30].

Notably, in a subsequent study by Cipriano et al., examining 871 patients undergoing revision hip or knee surgery,

61 patients with known inflammatory arthritis were included [43]. In this study, the definition of PJI was based on a variation of the IDSA criteria. Specifically, patients were considered to have PJI if they had two of the following criteria: sinus tract, intraoperative purulence, one positive deep culture or histopathological findings consistent with infection [931, 43]. In this large cohort study, 165 patients met the above definition of PJI. Of interest, the optimal thresholds did not differ significantly between inflammatory and noninflammatory cases [43]. Overall a cut-off of 3450 leucocyte count/μL had a sensitivity of 91% (95% confidence interval 81–94%) and a specificity of 93% (95% confidence interval 91–95%). Similarly, applying a cut-off of 78% for polymorphonuclear leucocyte percentage, the sensitivity was 95.5% (95% confidence interval 94–97%) and specificity 87% (85–90%) [43]. As with the serum inflammatory markers, in the previously described study by Bracken and colleagues, synovial leucocyte count and polymorphonuclear leucocyte percentage did not differ between bacterial and fungal infections [35]. Incorporating these findings, the new MSIS criteria cut-offs for chronic infections (defined as greater than 90 days of implantation) include a synovial leucocyte count of 3000 cells/μL and a polymorphonuclear leucocyte percentage of 80% [3].

As with other diagnostic tests, there are a number of limitations that hamper the utility of synovial fluid aspirate characteristics; firstly, thresholds are based on data from lower limb arthroplasty with little data to guide upper limb PJI diagnosis [31]. Secondly, metal-on-metal prosthesis failure falsely elevates the synovial cell count due to the presence of cellular debris when automated cell counts are performed. In a retrospective study Yi and colleagues examined 150 patients undergoing hip revision surgery with a metal-on-metal bearing surface or corrosion reaction [46]. Of the 141 synovial samples submitted for examination, the automated cell count was inaccurate in 33% due to the presence of metal debris and fragmented cells. The authors recommended that, in this setting, a manual cell count should be performed [46].

3.5   Other Synovial Fluid Biomarkers

3.5.1   Synovial Fluid Leucocyte Esterase

In recent years, there has been intense interest in investigating new biomarkers of PJI (Table 3.7) [1–3, 47–64]. One simple, commonly available marker, leucocyte esterase, has been investigated by a number of research groups. Leucocyte esterase is an enzyme released by neutrophils and other granulocytic leucocytes in the setting of infection [47]. This enzyme has been incorporated into urine reagent strip tests for the detection of urinary tract infections ("urine dipsticks") [47]. This test was adapted as a "point-of-care" test for the presence of leucocyte esterase in synovial fluid specimens. In an early report by Parvizi et al., intraoperative synovial samples from 108 patients undergoing revision knee arthroplasty were tested [47]. Applying a reading of "++", leucocyte esterase had a sensitivity of 80.6% (95% confidence interval 61.9–91.9%) and specificity of 100% (95% confidence interval 94.5–100%) [47]. When a cut-off of "+" or "++" was applied, the sensitivity increased to 93.5% (95% confidence interval 77.2–98.8%); however, this was to the detriment of specificity (86.7%; 95% confidence interval 77.1–92.9%) [47]. Expectedly, leucocyte esterase strongly correlated with synovial fluid leucocyte count ($r^2 = 0.78$) [47]. A subsequent study by Wetters et al. of 223 revision hip and knee arthroplasties applied a reading of "+" or "++"; when combined with a synovial fluid leucocyte count of greater than 3000 cells/μL, the sensitivity was 92.9% and specificity 88.8% [48]. In contrast to the earlier publication by Parvizi and colleagues, in the study by Wetters et al., a separate analysis examining a cut-off of "++" alone was not performed [48]. Similar results have been reported by other groups, including in the setting of metallosis [49–57, 66, 67]. It is important to note, however, that the performance of the colorimetric test is impaired or unreadable in the presence of excess red blood cells or cellular debris, which occurred in up to 30% of subjects in the reported literature [47, 48, 66].

TABLE 3.7 Selected literature review of test performance for synovial fluid biomarkers

Biomarker Reference	Joint(s)	Chronicity[a]	Number[b]	Threshold	Prosthetic joint infection criteria	Sensitivity (%)	Specificity (%)
Leukocyte esterase							
Parvizi et al. [47]	Knee	Not specified	108	"+" or "++"	*One or more of the following:* 1. Sinus tract 2. Intraoperative purulence 3. Positive cultures 4. Elevated serum biomarkers	93.5	87
Wetters et al. [48]	Knee and hip	Not specified	223	"+" or "++" (and synovial fluid leukocyte count >3000 cells/ μL)	Organism isolated from ≥2 cultures *or two of the following:* 1. Sinus tract 2. Intraoperative purulence 3. Organism isolated from 1 culture 4. Histology consistent with infection	93	89

Shafafy et al. [49]	Knee and hip	Not specified	109	"++"	Osmon et al. [1] IDSA criteria	82	93
De Vecchi et al. [50]	Knee and hip	Not specified	129	"+" or "++"	Parvizi and Gehrke [3] revised MSIS criteria	93	97
Deirmengian et al. [51]	Knee and hip	Not specified	46	"++"	Original MSIS criteria [2]	69	100
Colvin et al. [52]	Knee, hip, and shoulder	Not specified	52	"++"	*One or more of the following*: 1. Positive culture results *and* white blood cell count >1700 cells/μL 2. Positive culture results *and* elevated polymorphonuclear cell percentage > 65% 3. Intraoperative purulence	100	97
Nelson et al. [53]	Shoulder	Not specified	16	"+" or "++"	Original MSIS criteria [2]	25	75

(continued)

TABLE 3.7 (continued)

Biomarker	Reference	Joint(s)	Chronicity[a]	Number[b]	Threshold	Prosthetic joint infection criteria	Sensitivity (%)	Specificity (%)
Synovial C-reactive protein (CRP)								
	Deirmengian et al. [54]	Knee and hip	Not specified	95	12.2 mg/L	Original MSIS criteria [2]	90	97
	De Vecchi et al. [50]	Knee and hip	Not specified	129	10 mg/L	Parvizi and Gehrke [3] revised MSIS criteria	82	94
	Parvizi et al. [55]	Knee and hip	Not specified	63 patients (55 undergoing revision arthroplasty)	9.5 mg/L	Three of the following: 1. ESR >30 mm/h 2. Serum CRP >10 mg/L 3. Synovial white cell count ≥1760 cells/μL for chronic infection or >10,700 cells/μL for acute infection 4. Synovial polymorph percentage > 73% for chronic infection or >89% for acute infection	85	95

Study	Joint	Chronicity	N	CRP cutoff	Criteria	Sensitivity	Specificity
Tetreault et al. [56]	Knee and hip	Not specified	119	6.6 mg/L	Modified original MSIS criteria [2]: serum CRP excluded from criteria	88	85
Omar et al. [57]	Hip	Chronic (>6 weeks)	89	9.5 mg/L	*One or more of the following:* 1. Sinus tract 2. Purulent synovial fluid 3. Positive cultures 4. *Three of the following:* (a) ESR > 30 mm/h (b) Serum CRP > 10 mg/L (c) Synovial white cell count >1760 cells/μL (d) Synovial polymorph percentage >73%	95.5	93
Alpha-defensin							
Deirmengian et al. [51]	Knee and hip	Not specified	46	5.2 mg/L	Original MSIS criteria [2]	100	100

(continued)

TABLE 3-7 (continued)

Biomarker	Reference	Joint(s)	Chronicity[a]	Number[b]	Threshold	Prosthetic joint infection criteria	Sensitivity (%)	Specificity (%)
	Bonanzinga et al. [58]	Knee and hip	Not specified	156	Signal-to-cut-off ratio 1.0	Parvizi and Gehrke [3] revised MSIS criteria	97	97
	Deirmengian et al. [59]	Knee and hip	Not specified	149	Signal-to-cut-off ratio 1.0	Original MSIS criteria [2]	97	95.5
	Deirmengian et al. [54]	Knee and hip	Not specified	95	4.8μg/L	Original MSIS criteria [2]	100	100
	Frangiamore et al. [60]	Knee and hip	Not specified	116	5.2 mg/L	Original MSIS criteria [2]	100	98
	Bingham et al. [61]	Knee and hip	Not specified	51	7720 ng/mL	Original MSIS criteria [2]	100	95
	Kasparek et al. [62]	Knee and hip	Chronic (>90 days)	40	Positive lateral flow test	Parvizi and Gehrke [3] revised MSIS criteria	67	93

			Parvizi and Gehrke [3] revised MSIS criteria	69	94
Sigmund et al. [63]	Knee, hip, shoulder, and elbow	Not specified	Positive lateral flow test	50	
Frangiamore et al. [64]	Shoulder	Not specified	Organism isolated from ≥2 cultures	63	95
			Signal-to-cut-off ratio 0.48	33	

[a]Unless otherwise specified, chronicity refers to the time from index prosthetic joint surgery until prosthetic joint revision surgery

[b]Number of revision arthroplasties

ISDA Infectious Diseases Society of America, *MSIS* Musculoskeletal Infection Society, *ESR* erythrocyte sedimentation rate

An intermediate centrifugation step has been suggested as a potential mechanism to overcome this issue; however, this is not in keeping with the original ethos of the test being a "point-of-care" test [50, 66]. The test performance is decreased in shoulder arthroplasties as noted by Nelson and colleagues in a study of 16 revision shoulder arthroplasties [53]. *C. acnes* was isolated from ten patients in this cohort. Overall, the sensitivity of leucocyte esterase was 25.0% and the specificity was 75.0%. In the patients from whom *C. acnes* was isolated, the sensitivity was only 18.2% [53]. Despite these uncertainties, a "+" or "++" change on leucocyte esterase test strip has been incorporated as a minor criterion in the revised MSIS criteria [3].

3.5.2   Synovial Fluid CRP

In further studies published by Deirmengian and colleagues, a number of synovial fluid biomarkers were identified as potential aids in PJI diagnosis [54, 68]. In an early study involving 95 patients undergoing prosthetic hip or knee revision surgery, including 29 PJI classified according to the original MSIS criteria, five biomarkers were noted to have a high sensitivity (100%; 95% confidence interval 88–100%, respectively) and high specificity (100%; 95% confidence interval 95–100%, respectively): human α-defensin, neutrophil elastase 2, bactericidal/permeability-increasing protein, neutrophil gelatinase-associated lipocalin and lactoferrin [54]. In addition, synovial CRP was noted to have a sensitivity of 90% (95% confidence interval 73–98%) and specificity 97% (95% confidence interval 90–100%) [54].

Given that serum CRP assay is widely available, Parvizi et al. built on this early biomarker work, to further examine the potential role of synovial fluid CRP as a diagnostic test for PJI [65]. The performance of synovial fluid CRP using two assays was assessed in a small prospective study involving 66 patients undergoing revision knee arthroplasty. Diagnosis of PJI was based on the institutional definition which included the presence of sinus tract, intraoperative purulence, positive periprosthetic tissue or fluid culture or any of the following: ESR ≥ 30 mm/h, CRP ≥10 mg/L or synovial leucocyte count ≥1760 cells/lL or synovial fluid polymorphonuclear leucocyte percent ≥73% [65]. The test performance of the individual and the multiplex ELISA were similar with sensitivities of 70.0% and 84.0% and specificities of 100.0% and 97.1%, respectively. Of note, there was no statistically significant difference between synovial fluid and serum CRP values [65].

Subsequently, Parvizi and colleagues further examined the role of synovial CRP in 55 patients undergoing revision hip or knee arthroplasty [55]. The cohort also included eight patients undergoing primary knee joint replacement. In contrast to the early study, the diagnosis of PJI was made purely on the basis of inflammatory markers or synovial fluid characteristics, with the diagnosis of PJI considered if three of the following were present: ESR greater than 30 mm/h, a serum CRP value greater than 10 mg/L, a synovial fluid leucocyte count greater than 1760 cells/µL for chronic infection or 10,700 cells/µL for acute infection or a synovial fluid polymorphonuclear leucocyte percent greater than 73% for chronic infection or greater than 89% for acute infection [55]. Based on this definition, 20 patients met these criteria for PJI. The synovial fluid CRP was significantly higher in patients with PJI; however, the synovial fluid CRP strongly correlated with the serum CRP ($r^2 = 0.72$) [55]. Applying a cut-off of 9.5 mg/L, the synovial fluid CRP had a sensitivity of 85% and specificity of 95.2% [55]. In a second study by Omar et al., a lower cut-off value for synovial fluid CRP of 2.5 mg/L was applied, and the authors reported a sensitivity of 95.5% (95% confidence interval 86.7–99.9%) and specificity of 93.3% (95% confidence interval 84.3–99.9%) in chronic hip PJI [57]. The authors noted that the performance of synovial fluid CRP was superior to serum CRP; however, it should be noted that the 95% confidence intervals for both tests overlapped; therefore, there was no statistical evidence to support a difference [57]. In a subsequent publication by Tetreault et al., evaluating 150 patients undergoing hip or knee arthroplasty revision, serum and synovial CRP were strongly correlated ($r^2 = 0.76$) [56].

There is evidence to suggest that CRP may be manufactured at sites other than the liver; however, there is no current evidence that CRP is manufactured de novo in the synovium [60, 69]. Parvizi et al. postulated the elevated synovial fluid CRP may reflect transmigration of the protein from the serum into the synovial space, particularly in the setting of inflammation [55]. In a recent publication by Deirmengian et al. examining 21,421 stored synovial fluids samples, it was noted that infections with organisms classified as "less virulent" such as *S. epidermidis* and yeast had lower mean synovial fluid CRP values than when compared to infections with more "virulent" organisms (15.10 vs. 32.70 mg/L; $P < 0.0001$) [70]. Overall, the utility of synovial fluid CRP, particularly over and above serum CRP, has not been established, and it has not been incorporated into diagnostic algorithms to date.

3.5.3   Synovial Fluid α-Defensin

In recent years, there has been increasing focus on α-defensin. α-Defensin is an antimicrobial peptide produced by the innate immune system [71]. In a study by Deirmengian et al. of 149 patients with hip or knee joint replacements, synovial fluid α-defensin had a sensitivity of 97.3% (95% confidence interval 85.5–99.6%) and a specificity of 95.5% (95% confidence interval 89.9–98.5%) [59]. Patients with metallosis, inflammatory arthritis and prior antibiotic therapy were not specifically excluded in this study, and the presence of these factors did not impact the test performance of α-defensin, similarly to other reports [59, 72]. When combined with synovial fluid CRP, the authors reported the specificity improved to 100% (95% confidence interval 96.7–100%) and sensitivity 97.3% (95% confidence intervals 85.8–99.6%) [59]. The authors applied the original MSIS criteria for PJI, which includes elevated CRP as a minor criterion: therefore, this may introduce circularity given the correlation between serum and synovial CRP and the incorporation of this marker into the definition for this study [59]. Further studies by this research group have demonstrated that the test performance of α-defensin is preserved in infections caused by a wide range of microorganisms including "less virulent" microorganisms [73]. However, as with other diagnostic tests, in shoulder arthroplasty infections, α-defensin does not perform as well. In a study by Frangiamore et al., the sensitivity of α-defensin was 63% with preserved specificity (95%) [64, 74]. In a recent meta-analysis by Wyatt et al., incorporating the above studies, the combined sensitivity of α-defensin was 100% (95% confidence interval 82–100%) and specificity 96% (95% confidence interval 89–99%) [75]. Significant heterogeneity was noted amongst the included studies, and, as noted by the authors, a number of studies came from the same research group [75]. Further studies published subsequent to the meta-analysis report lower sensitivities including a study by Kasparek and colleagues examining chronic infections where the reported sensitivity was 67% (95% confidence interval 35–89%) [62]. Similarly in a study by Sigmund and colleagues, the sensitivity of α-defensin (69%; 95% confidence interval 46–92%) did not differ significantly from frozen section (73%; 95% confidence interval 46–100%), microbiological culture with ≥ two positive cultures (85%; 95% confidence interval 62–100%) or serum C-reactive protein (77%; 95% confidence interval 54–100%) [63]. The data from α-defensin is promising; however, wider validation across a range of clinical scenarios is required. There is no data on the cost or cost-effectiveness of this test, nor on the optimal clinical setting for testing, including whether the test should be performed in all infections, acute or chronic PJI.

3.6 Radiological Studies

3.6.1 Plain Radiographs

Plain radiographs are commonly performed in patients presenting with prosthesis failure [4]. These tests, however, lack sensitivity and specificity in diagnosing PJI as findings such as lucency around the prosthesis can be noted in both septic and aseptic loosening [76–79]. In an early study reported by Duff and colleagues, focal osteolysis was observed in 36% and 38%

of infected and noninfected knee arthroplasties, respectively, at the time of revision [77]. Similarly in hip arthroplasties, in a study by Cyteval et al., there was no radiographic abnormality detected in 25% of infected compared to 28% of noninfected prosthetic hips [76]. The sensitivity of focal lucency was poor (25%) with moderate specificity (79%) [76]. In addition, there is a lag in the time from onset of infection until the development of radiographic changes [78].

3.6.2   Radionuclide Bone Scintigraphy

Radionuclide imaging techniques such as radionuclide bone scintigraphy have a high reported negative predictive value (reported by Smith et al. as 95.0%); however, they lack specificity, particularly to distinguish septic from aseptic failure [76, 80]. In addition, bone scans can remain positive for a year following uncomplicated arthroplasty [76, 80]. Similar findings and limitations have been documented with newer modalities such as [18]fluorodeoxyglucose-positron emission tomography ([18]FDG-PET) [81, 82]. A meta-analysis of [18]FDG-PET, including 11 studies, reported a sensitivity for hip PJI of 82.1% (95% confidence interval 68.0–90.8%) and for knee PJI of 86.6% (95% confidence interval 79.7–91.4%) [83]. The authors noted that the specificity of [18]FDG-PET was significantly higher for hip PJI compared to knee PJI (89.8% versus 74.8%) [83]. At the recent Consensus Meeting on Periprosthetic Joint Infection, the high cost of these tests and lack of cost-effectiveness data were highlighted as a limitation for the incorporation of radionuclide imaging into current diagnostic algorithms [4].

3.6.3   Computed Tomography and Magnetic Resonance Imaging

In the study by Cyteval et al. including 63 patients with painful hip prostheses, computed tomography (CT) was useful in detecting abnormalities of the soft tissues, in particular "joint distension" with a sensitivity of 83% and specificity of 96%; however, CT scans did not perform as well for differentiation between periprosthetic bone abnormalities due to aseptic and septic loosening, with a sensitivity of 75% and a poor specificity of 30% [76]. Magnetic resonance imaging is also of limited value in the diagnosis of PJI as artefact from the prosthesis impedes interpretation [4, 16, 79, 84].

3.7   Microbiological Culture

The isolation of an identical microorganism (or microorganisms) from two or more aseptically obtained periprosthetic specimens is a major criterion for infection, regardless of definition applied [1–4]. In addition to confirmation of infection, microbiological cultures enable antimicrobial susceptibility testing to guide treatment and prevention decisions. As with other areas of PJI diagnosis, a number of questions exist including which specimen(s) should be obtained, the optimal method of specimen collection, the optimal number of specimens to be collected to maximise diagnosis, the media used for microbiological culture, the best methods for species identification of microorganisms and how long culture should be incubated. Many of the questions have been examined in recent research.

3.7.1   Synovial Fluid and Synovium Biopsy Culture

In addition to the valuable information about the cellular profile, synovial fluid aspiration allows for microbiological culture of the specimen with preoperative identification of the pathogen to aid with preoperative surgery and antimicrobial decisions. In a meta-analysis by Qu et al., the sensitivity of synovial aspirate culture was 72% (95% confidence interval 65–78%) with good specificity (95%; 95% confidence interval 93–97%). In this study, there was marked heterogeneity in definitions, and there was no information on culture methods or duration of cultures [85]. Of relevance, studies have demonstrated increased yields when synovial fluid is inoculated and culture performed in blood culture bottles, compared with conventional plate and broth culture techniques [86]. In addition, the sensitivity of synovial aspirate culture differs between acute and chronic infections: Font-Vizcarra et al. demonstrated a significant difference in sensitivity for the culture of synovial fluid between acute and chronic infections (91% versus 79%, respectively) [87].

A number of studies have investigated whether performing preoperative synovial biopsy has increased sensitivity compared to synovial fluid aspiration: in a study by Fink et al. examining 145 patients undergoing total knee revision, synovial biopsy had a sensitivity of 77.5% (95% confidence interval 64.6–90.4%) which was similar to aspiration (sensitivity 72.5%; 95% confidence interval 58.7–86.3%) with a specificity of 98.1% (95% confidence interval 95.5–100%) compared to 95.2% (95% confidence interval 91.2–99.2%), respectively [88]. When the biopsy culture was combined with histological examination, the sensitivity increased to 100% [88]. In a similar study in 273 patients undergoing revision hip arthroplasty, the sensitivity of aspiration did not differ significantly from biopsy (80% versus 83%, respectively) with similar specificity (94% versus 90%, respectively) [89]. Therefore, at present, there is no clear benefit of synovial biopsy over aspiration, particularly as synovial biopsy is a more invasive procedure [89].

3.7.2 Optimal Specimen Type

A study by Tetreault et al., comparing superficial culture of draining wounds or sinus tracts to periprosthetic samples in 55 patients, demonstrated poor concordance between the culture specimens [90]. Less than half of superficial cultures were concordant with periprosthetic cultures (47.3%; 95% confidence interval 34.7–60.2%) with an increase preponderance of polymicrobial culture results obtained with superficial cultures (43.4%) [90]. The authors commented that, if the superficial cultures had been acted upon, this would have resulted in alteration in the antimicrobial regimen selected in 41.8% of cases, including the addition of antimicrobials in 20% of cases [90]. Overall, the authors concluded that superficial culture of draining wounds or sinus tracts should be discouraged [90].

Intraoperatively, the optimal method of specimen collection was recently studied by Aggarwal and colleagues [91]. In a prospective study involving 156 patients, the performance of tissue and swab intraoperative specimens for microbiological culture was compared. Overall, tissue culture was superior to swab cultures with an increased sensitivity (93% versus 70%, respectively) and increased specificity (98% versus 89%) [91]. The rate of contamination of specimens was higher with swabs compared to tissue culture (12% versus 2%, respectively; $P = 0.032$) [91]. The authors concluded that the collection of intraoperative swabs of microbiological culture should be avoided [91].

In a subsequent study by Bémer and colleagues, the optimal site of periprosthetic tissue sampling was examined [92]. This multicentre, prospective study included patients with clinical suspicion of PJI; all patients had six samples collected—five for culture and 16S rRNA gene PCR and one for histological examination. Diagnosis of PJI was based on modified IDSA criteria, with the exclusion of intraoperative purulence; of note, bacteriological criteria were included in the PJI definition [92]. Applying this definition, 215 patients were classified as having PJI. Bémer and colleagues noted that samples taken from tissue in contact with the prosthetic material and synovial fluids samples had the highest rate of positivity (91.5% and 91.7%, respectively), whereas cancellous bone had the lowest rate of positivity (76.6%) [92].

3.7.3   Optimal Number of Specimens

Given that diagnostic criteria include the isolation of the same microorganism(s) on two or more periprosthetic specimens, it stands to reason that two or more periprosthetic specimens must be obtained for culture [1–3]. Until recently, there was limited data on the number of specimens required for optimal diagnostic yield. An early study by Atkins and colleagues investigated a number of aspects of microbiological diagnosis, including the optimal number of specimens required for PJI diagnosis [93]. The diagnosis of PJI was based on histological characteristics defined as the presence of five or more neutrophils per high-power field [93]. As an initial aim, Atkins and colleagues examined the post-test probability of PJI with increasing numbers of specimens isolating the same microorganism. A single positive culture had a low post-test probability of infection (10.6%), increasing to 80.6% when the same microorganism was isolated on two or more specimens, and was highest when the same microorganism was isolated from three or more specimens (96.4%); the isolation of the same microorganisms in three or more specimens had a sensitivity of 66% and a specificity of 99.6% [93]. Applying mathematical modelling, the number of specimens needed to isolate the same organism on three or more specimens was greater than seven specimens [93]. The authors suggested that the collection and culturing of seven specimens was likely to pose challenges for the clinical microbiology laboratory and would be impractical. Applying the same model, the collection of five to six specimens isolating the same microorganisms from two or more specimens was associated with a similar sensitivity, to the minor detriment of the specificity, when compared to the isolation of three or more indistinguishable organisms (exact values not provided in the publication) [93]. The authors concluded that five to six intraoperative specimens of periprosthetic tissue and a cut-off of two or more specimens isolating the same organism were reasonable for the diagnosis of PJI [93]. Atkins and colleagues also highlighted that routine Gram staining of periprosthetic tissue had a very low sensitivity (12%), and the authors discouraged Gram staining for detection of PJI at revision arthroplasty [93].

Marín et al. applied the same methodology as Atkins et al. to examine the optimal number of specimens comparing microbiological culture to 16S RNA PCR [94]. At variance with Atkins et al., PJI was defined if there was evidence of periprosthetic purulence and histological features of inflammation or if a sinus tract was present. Overall, 122 patients were included in the study, 40 of whom met the definition for PJI. Microbiological culture had a higher sensitivity (75.9%; 95% confidence interval 68.8–81.9%) compared to 16S RNA PCR (67.1%; 95% confidence interval 59.7–73.6%); however, the specificity was lower (81.2% [95% confidence interval 76.7–85.0%] versus 97.8% [95% confidence interval 95.6–98.9%], respectively) [94]. In keeping with the findings by Atkins et al., the isolation of the same microorganism in three or more specimens when five samples were cultured had a sensitivity of 80% and specificity of 96.8% [94]. Correspondingly, performing 16S ribosomal RNA (rRNA) gene PCR on five specimens and isolating the same microorganism in two or more specimens were associated with a sensitivity of 94% and specificity of 100% [94].

In the previously mentioned study by Bémer and colleagues, in addition to examining optimal sampling site, these authors revisited the question of the optimal number of specimens required for PJI diagnosis [92]. The authors compared the agreement between IDSA criteria for PJI and bacteriological criteria which included a single positive culture for "virulent microorganisms" such as *S. aureus*, Gram-negative bacilli or anaerobic organisms or two or more cultures for "skin commensals" such as coagulase-negative staphylococci or *C. acnes* [92]. The authors noted that the mean percentage agreement for PJI diagnosis was similar with three samples (99.2%; 95% confidence interval 98.4–100.0%) compared to four samples (99.7%; 95% confidence interval 99.0–100.0%). The percentage agreement for the bacteriological criterion was higher with four samples (98.1%;

95% confidence interval 96.4–99.5%) compared to three samples (93.9%; 95% confidence interval 91.1–96.4%). The authors recommended, therefore, that four samples be obtained [92].

These results are similar to a study by Peel et al., which compared periprosthetic tissue culture using conventional methods with inoculation of tissue specimens into blood culture bottles. This large prospective study included 499 patients undergoing revision arthroplasty for septic and aseptic failure. The diagnosis of PJI was based on the modified IDSA criteria whereby the microbiological criterion was excluded to avoid circularity [95]. Applying Bayesian latent class modelling, the greatest accuracy was observed when four periprosthetic tissue samples were cultured using conventional culture techniques (accuracy 91%; 95% credible interval 77–100%). In contrast, the greatest accuracy was observed when three periprosthetic tissue specimens were inoculated into blood culture bottles (accuracy 92%; 95% credible interval 79–100%; Fig. 3.2) [95].

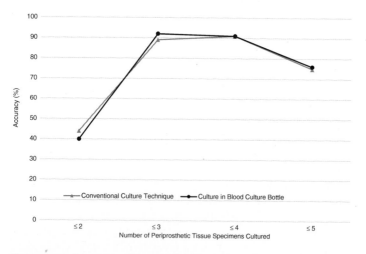

FIGURE 3.2 Accuracy of conventional periprosthetic tissue cultures versus culture in blood culture bottles. Based on data from Peel et al. [95]

3.7.4   Optimal Culture Media

There are limited studies examining the optimal media for culturing periprosthetic tissue biopsies [31]. Conventional microbiological techniques frequently include culture on various types of aerobic and anaerobic agar plates and inoculation into broths; however, these methods are not standardised and differ across different laboratories [31, 93, 96]. A recent study by Hughes and colleagues compared four different tissue culture techniques in 141 subjects including culture on blood and chocolate agars, in Robertson's cooked meat broth, in fastidious anaerobic broth and in aerobic and anaerobic blood culture bottles [96]. The authors defined PJI on the basis of histopathological findings with 23 subjects meeting this criterion [96]. Blood culture bottles were more sensitive compared to direct tissue culture and fastidious anaerobic broth (87% [95% confidence intervals 72–100%] vs. 39% [95% confidence intervals 18–61%], $P = 0.007$, and 57% [95% confidence intervals 35–78%], $P = 0.016$, respectively) [96]. There was no difference in sensitivity between culture in blood culture bottles and cooked meat broth (83% [95% confidence intervals 66–99%]; $P = 0.74$) [96].

A second study by Peel and colleagues compared the test performance of aerobic and anaerobic agars, thioglycolate broth and aerobic and anaerobic blood culture bottles. The study included 369 consecutive subjects undergoing revision arthroplasty, of which 117 (32%) met IDSA criteria for PJI [1, 6]. Analysing individual media, for aerobic culture, inoculation of periprosthetic tissue in aerobic blood culture bottles was associated with improved sensitivity when compared to aerobic agar culture (sensitivity 82.0%; 95% credible interval 69.5–91.1% versus 59.4%; 95% credible interval 45.3–72.5%) [6]. Similarly, anaerobic culture in anaerobic blood culture bottles was more sensitive than anaerobic agar and thioglycolate broth cultures (sensitivity 90.2%; 95% credible interval 79.4–96.5% versus 32.2%; 95% credible interval 20.8–45.7% and 74.8%;

95% credible interval 61.5–85.8%) [6]. When examining combinations of media, the combination of culture in aerobic and anaerobic blood culture bottles was associated with increased sensitivity compared to conventional agar and broth cultures applying Bayesian latent class modelling (92.1% [95% credible interval 84.9–97.0%] vs. 62.6% [95% credible interval 51.7–72.5%], respectively) [6]. The specificity of culture in blood culture bottles was similar to culture using conventional media [6]. Therefore, both studies support the inoculation of periprosthetic tissue specimens into blood culture bottles to improve the diagnostic yield of microbiological culture [6, 96].

In addition to the optimal number of specimens required for PJI diagnosis, a further aim of the study by Bémer and colleagues was to examine the optimal culture media for PJI diagnosis [92]. Periprosthetic tissue specimens were inoculated onto/into blood agar and chocolate agar incubated for 7 days aerobically, a blood agar incubated anaerobically for 7 days, a paediatric blood culture bottle incubated for 14 days and Schaedler broth incubated for 14 days. With respect to anaerobic culture methods, the authors noted that Schaedler broth was superior to blood agar cultured anaerobically, yielding a microorganism in 72.5% of specimens compared to 56.2%, respectively [92]. The potential impact of the difference in incubation times between the two media was not specifically commented on by the authors. With respect to aerobic culture methods, paediatric blood culture bottles yielded 83% of identified aerobes, higher when compared with blood agar (70.1%), chocolate agar (69.0%) and Schaedler broth (68.8%) [92]. Overall, Bémer and colleagues suggested optimal results were obtained when periprosthetic tissue samples were inoculated onto a combination of blood culture bottle, chocolate agar and Schaedler broth [92]. At variance with the study by Peel et al., anaerobic blood culture bottles were not inoculated; also, the study by Bémer et al. involved only patients with suspected or proven PJI, therefore limiting further comparison [6, 92].

3.7.5 Microorganism Identification

The optimal method for identification and species identification of microorganisms should also be considered; given the costs associated with species identification of bacteria, many laboratories historically only reported identifications to the genus level for many bacteria including coagulase-negative *Staphylococcus* species and *Corynebacterium* species [97, 98]. With the advent of matrix-assisted laser desorption-ionisation time-of-flight mass spectrometry (MALDI-TOF MS), rapid and accurate identification of bacteria to the species level is possible in routine clinical practice for the diagnosis of PJI [98, 99]. Given that current IDSA and MSIS definitions for periprosthetic tissue infection include isolation of the same microorganisms from two or more specimens, the ability to confirm species improves diagnostic certainty [1–3]. In an early study by Harris and colleagues, the authors examined the ability of MALDI-TOF MS to identify staphylococci isolates from PJI cases [97]. The study involved 79 strain pairs of staphylococci which included *S. aureus*, *S. epidermidis*, *Staphylococcus capitis*, *Staphylococcus lugdunensis*, *Staphylococcus haemolyticus* and *Staphylococcus warneri* [97]. These isolates had been originally characterised by clumping factor and API ID32 STAPH (BioMerieux, Marcy l'Etoile, France) [97]. MALDI-TOF MS correctly identified all isolates [97].

As a second aim of the study, Harris and colleagues assessed the ability of MALDI-TOF MS to subtype four reference strains of *S. epidermidis* [97]. The authors found that MALDI Biotyper software was also able to correctly subtype *S. epidermidis* strains [97]. This may assist in assessment of whether isolates are clonally related, which will guide epidemiological and infection control investigations [97].

In addition, in a descriptive study by Peel and colleagues, examining 770 clinical isolates from periprosthetic tissue and fluid samples, there was the suggestion that the profile of staphylococcal species that were associated with infection compared to contamination differed [98]. Organisms such as *S. aureus* and *Staphylococcus caprae* were always pathogens, isolated into two or more specimens in patients meeting the IDSA criteria for PJI, compared to *Staphylococcus pasteuri* and *Staphylococcus pettenkoferi* which were contaminants, being isolated only in a single specimen in patients otherwise not meeting the criteria for infection. Given the small size of this sample, definitive differences could not be characterised; however, this observation may be confirmed with the ongoing development of MALDI-TOF MS organism databases and larger studies [98]. Of further relevance, given the increasing number of studies examining the role of culture of periprosthetic tissue specimens in blood culture bottles, MALDI-TOF MS can be performed directly from blood culture bottles, therefore improving the rapidity of identification [98].

3.7.6   Culture Duration

It is recognised that growth time differs between different microorganisms; in particular, *C. acnes* is considered a slow grower with prolonged doubling times [100, 101]. Prolongation of microbiological culture incubation duration, therefore, may help to improve the diagnostic yield. An early study by Schäfer and colleagues examined optimal culture duration and included 284 patients undergoing revision arthroplasty [101]. Patients were diagnosed with PJI if the same microorganism was isolated in two or more specimens or if a single culture was positive in a patient with histopathological features consistent with infection. Thereby, 110 specimens originated from patients meeting the definition of PJI, and 47 specimens were considered contaminants [101]. In the patients meeting the definition for PJI, 73.6% of infections were diagnosed within the first 7 days. However, over one quarter of infections were diagnosed in the second week of culture and would have been missed if culture duration was not extended to 14 days [101]. Conversely, 52% of contaminating organisms were cultured within the first week of culture [101]. Extending incubation of periprosthetic tissue culture to 14 days improved detection of microorganisms such as *Cutibacterium* species, *Peptostreptococcus* species and coryneform bacteria; many of these microorganisms would not have been detected if cultures had only been incubated for 7 days [101].

Butler-Wu et al. also examined the optimal duration for PJI due to *C. acnes* [100]. This study included 87 revision arthroplasties, the majority of which were shoulder arthroplasty revisions (83%) [100]. Tissue specimens were cultured on blood, chocolate and brucella agar in addition to brain heart infusion broth. Infection was confirmed either on the basis of isolation of the same microorganism in two or more specimens or, in the event of a single positive culture, if histology was suggestive of infection. Based on these criteria, infection was diagnosed in 42 revision arthroplasties, including 23 cases where *C. acnes* was isolated [100]. The authors identified the optimal duration of culture incubation to be 13 days. Extending culture durations beyond 13 days was associated with increased isolation of contaminants [100]. In addition, Butler-Wu et al. recommended that both the anaerobic and aerobic cultures should be extended: in 29.4% of *C. acnes* PJI cases, the diagnosis would have been missed if only the anaerobic culture duration had been extended [100].

Minassian and colleagues examined duration of culture for periprosthetic tissue specimens inoculated into anaerobic and aerobic blood culture bottles [102]. The study included 332 patients undergoing revision arthroplasty for suspected PJI with infection confirmed in 79, according to the IDSA criteria [102]. The majority of blood culture bottles were positive within 3 days of incubation; however, *Cutibacterium* species was isolated after a median of 5-day incubation (range 3 to 13 days). No clinically significant microorganism was isolated with terminal subculture of blood culture bottles after 14 days of incubation [102]. Minassian et al. concluded that prolonged culture for 14 days was not indicated, suggesting an optimal duration of 4-day incubation based on receiver operating characteristic analysis [102].

Similarly in the previously described study by Peel et al., the majority of organisms were isolated within 2 days of culture [6]. Extending blood culture bottle incubation beyond 7 days yielded three additional PJI diagnoses, all infections due to *Cutibacterium* species [6]. Conversely extending anaerobic blood culture bottle incubation beyond 7 days also yielded three contaminants, all *C. acnes* [6]. Therefore, studies examining duration of culture for periprosthetic tissue specimens inoculated into blood culture bottles suggest that shorter durations of culture may be reasonable. The caveat may relate to clinical scenarios where *C. acnes* is a common causative agent, such as with shoulder arthroplasty infections, in which case, extending cultures of blood culture bottles up to 14 days may improve diagnostic yield.

3.7.7   Sonicate Fluid Culture

The presence of biofilm is postulated as a contributory factor to the reduced sensitivity of culture of periprosthetic tissue culture with conventional culture techniques. Sonication of the prosthesis and subsequent culture of the sonicate fluid was developed in attempt to disrupt the biofilm and increase the yield of cultures. The technique applied differs between centres; however, in general, this process entails the application of mild sonication (40–50 Hz) to a resected prosthesis bathed in fluid [103, 104]. This fluid is then cultured and the number of colonies isolated is quantified (Fig. 3.3). With appropriate cut-offs for positivity, this technique may be used to confirm PJI based on a single sample, as opposed to periprosthetic tissue culture, where multiple samples must be positive to confirm diagnosis.

This technique was employed in early studies by Tunney et al. [103, 104]. It was further refined by Trampuz et al. in an early study of 78 patients undergoing revision hip or knee surgery [105]. A modified version of the IDSA criteria was applied (microbiological criteria were omitted) with 24 included patients meeting this definition [105]. The explanted

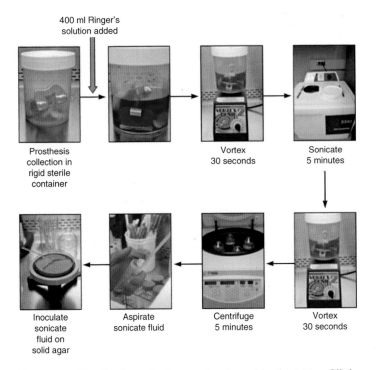

FIGURE 3.3 Prosthesis sonication protocol used in the Mayo Clinic Clinical Microbiology Laboratory [31] (©, Mayo Clinic, Rochester, MN, USA; courtesy of David T. Lynch, MT(ASCP), CLS(NCA])

prosthesis was placed in a sterile polyethylene bag, Ringer's solution was then added and sonication was performed. Of sonicate fluid, 0.5 mL was inoculated onto five aerobic and five anaerobic agars and cultured, and results were compared to results from standard tissue culture. Growth detected on any of the agar plates was considered as a significant result for the sonicate culture. Overall, culture of the sonicate culture was associated with an increased sensitivity (75%; 95% confidence interval 53–95%) compared to periprosthetic tissue culture in which the same microorganism was isolated on two or more specimens (sensitivity 54%; 95% confidence interval 33–75%) [105]. The authors found that there was a potential risk of contamination of the specimen with the use of the polyethylene bags [105].

In a follow-on study, the protocol was modified with polypropylene jars replacing the polyethylene bags used for prosthesis collection [106]. This modified protocol was then investigated in a larger prospective study of 331 patients undergoing revision hip or knee arthroplasty of whom 79 had PJI [106]. Aliquots of 0.5 mL of sonicate fluid were inoculated onto an aerobic and anaerobic sheep blood agar, and sonicate cultures were considered positive if at least five colonies of the same microorganisms were isolated on either plate [106]. Overall, sonication was more sensitive compared to periprosthetic tissue culture in which the same microorganism was cultured in two or more specimens (78.5% [95% confidence interval 67.8–86.9%] versus 60.8% [95% confidence interval 49.1–71.6%], respectively; $p < 0.001$) with a similar specificity (98.8% [95% confidence interval 96.6–99.8%] versus 99.2% [95% confidence interval 97.2–99.9%]) [106]. The authors noted that sonication was particularly useful in cases where patients had received antibiotics perioperatively [106]. If a patient had received antimicrobials in the 14 days prior to revision arthroplasty, the sensitivity for periprosthetic tissue culture (based on the isolation of an organism in one or more specimen) decreased from 76.9% to 45%, whereas the sensitivity for sonicate fluid culture decreased to 75% ($P < 0.001$) [106].

The same research group applied a similar protocol to examine sonication in shoulder arthroplasty revision [9]. This study by Piper and colleagues included 136 patients undergoing shoulder revision arthroplasty of whom 33 patients had definite PJI. Culture of the sonicate fluid yielded an additional four microbiological diagnosis compared to periprosthetic tissue culture techniques. The sensitivity and specificity for sonicate culture were 66.7% and 98.0%, respectively, compared to 54.5% and 95.1%, respectively, for periprosthetic tissue culture [9]. *C. acnes* was identified as the causative agent in almost 40% of cases of PJI; the authors did not comment on whether sonication culture improved the sensitivity for detection of *C. acnes* [9].

A recent meta-analysis was undertaken by Zhai et al. in which, in addition to the three studies discussed above, nine additional studies were included [107]. The studies included both upper and lower limb arthroplasty; however, the majority of data for upper limb arthroplasty were derived from the previously discussed study by Piper et al. [9, 107]. Overall, the studies were noted to be of moderate quality [107]. The pooled sensitivity of sonicate culture was 80% (95% confidence interval 74–84%) and specificity 95% (95% confidence interval 90–98%) [107]. The authors also performed subgroup analyses examining specific aspects of culture including specimen processing and culture duration. Extending anaerobic culture to 14 days was associated with increased sensitivity of 83% (95% confidence interval 74–89%) compared to 78% (95% confidence interval 69–85%) for 7 days for anaerobic sonicate culture; however, as the 95% confidence intervals overlapped, this was not significant. Similarly, applying a cut-off of ≥5, colony-forming units/mL was associated with the highest sensitivity (82%; 95% confidence interval 76–87%) compared to other cut-offs (≥1, ≥20 and ≥50 colony-forming units/mL); however, this was not significantly different [107].

The recent International Consensus Meeting on Periprosthetic Joint Infection recommended that sonication should not be routinely performed on all explanted prosthetic material but reserved for patients where preoperative synovial aspirates have failed to yield an organism or if the patient has received antibiotics in the 2 weeks prior to revision arthroplasty [4].

3.8   Molecular Techniques

Despite techniques such as sonication and use of blood culture bottles, current culture methods may fail to identify an organism in 5–10% of patients with PJI, particularly in the setting of recent antimicrobial exposure [14, 108]. Molecular techniques, such as polymerase chain reaction (PCR), have been investigated in an attempt to improve diagnostic yield. These molecular techniques apply either "broad-range PCR", such as bacterial 16S rRNA gene PCR, or species-specific PCR targeting a single organism or group or organisms, such as with panel PCR.

3.8.1   Broad-Range Bacterial 16S rRNA Gene PCR

A number of studies have investigated the role of broad-range bacterial 16S rRNA gene PCR. Early studies were hampered by a lack of clear definition of PJI [104, 109–115]. In the previously discussed study by Marín et al. involving 122 patients, the sensitivity of 16S rRNA PCR was non-significantly reduced (67.1%; 95% confidence interval 59.7–73.6%) compared to periprosthetic tissue culture (75.9%; 95% confidence interval 68.8–81.9%) [94]. However PCR was significantly more specific (97.8% [95% confidence interval 95.6–98.9%] versus 81.2% [95% confidence interval 76.7–85.0%]). This observation by Marín et al. is at odds with prior studies which reported low specificity and high false-positive results. A study by Clarke et al. compared 31 total hip revision arthroplasties to 28 control primary hip arthroplasty surgeries, all of whom had no clinical, biochemical or histological features of infection. Overall bacterial DNA was detected in 45.8% of the tissue specimens in patients undergoing revision arthroplasty; however, bacterial DNA was also detected in 21.4% of tissue specimens from patients undergoing primary joint replacement surgery [113]. The authors postulated that these cases where bacterial DNA was detected may represent specimen contamination [113]. Potentially, the observed difference in specificity between current and older studies may represent improvement in specimen collection and handling. In meta-analysis by Qu and colleagues, including 14 studies, 12 of which used 16S rRNA gene PCR, the pooled sensitivity was 86% (95% confidence interval 77–92%) with a pooled specificity of 91% (95% confidence interval 81–96%) [114]. The meta-analysis included a subgroup analysis comparing 16S rRNA gene PCR to species-specific or multiplex PCR which demonstrated lower sensitivity and specificity for 16S rRNA gene PCR on the forest plot provided; however, the 95% confidence intervals overlap, with no evidence to support superiority of one PCR technique over the other [114]. In addition to issues with contamination, the other major limitation of "broad-range" PCR is its inability to identify individual pathogens in polymicrobial infections, which may occur in up to a third of cases [14, 31].

3.8.2   Species-Specific or Multiplex PCR

As noted in the meta-analysis, there are few studies examining the role of species-specific or multiplex PCR. In an early study by Kobayashi et al., species-specific PCR was performed for methicillin-resistant *Staphylococcus* targeting the *mecA* gene [115]. Diagnosis of infection was based on clinical, biochemical and histological findings with 23 of the 36 included patients determined to be infected [115]. Methicillin-resistant staphylococci were cultured in eight cases, all of which were positive by PCR [115]. PCR was also positive in six other patients from whom no methicillin-resistant staphylococci were found in microbiological culture; they were designated by the authors as false-positive results. The overall reported sensitivity was 100% and specificity was 79% [115]. The second study included in the meta-analysis examined the role of multiplex PCR [116]. In this study, Portillo and colleagues examined the utility of a real-time multiplex PCR kit for detection of microorganisms in sonicate fluid specimens. The kit used (SeptiFast©, Roche Diagnostics, Indianapolis IN, USA) was originally developed for the identification of pathogen-associated bloodstream infections [116]. The definition of PJI applied in this study mirrored that used by

Trampuz et al. [105, 116]. Pathogens were defined based on culture of a microorganism in one or more periprosthetic tissue specimens for "virulent" organisms such as *S. aureus* or in two or more periprosthetic tissue specimens for "low virulent" organisms such as *C. acnes* [116]. Sonicate fluid cultures were considered significant if there were ≥50 colony-forming units/mL [116]. The criterion for significant multiplex PCR results was not defined. The study cohort comprised of 62 cases of aseptic failure and 24 cases that met the defined PJI criteria. The application of multiplex PCR to sonicate fluid specimen was associated with increased sensitivity compared to sonicate fluid culture; however, the 95% confidence intervals overlapped (96% [95% confidence interval 79–99%] and 71% [95% confidence interval 49–87%], respectively) [116]. There were nine discordant results when multiplex PCR was compared to culture. In one patient *C. acnes* was isolated in periprosthetic tissue but not sonicate culture and was not detected by multiplex PCR: of note, *C. acnes* is not included in the SeptiFast kit. In three patients, *S. aureus* was detected by multiplex PCR but not periprosthetic tissue or sonicate culture; however, these cases had had these organisms detected from periprosthetic samples within the prior month and were receiving directed antimicrobial therapy against this organism [116]. Whether this result represents detection of degrading bacterial genetic material from dead microorganisms compared to persistence of infection was not discussed by the authors.

A similar study was undertaken by Achermann et al. comparing SeptiFast© multiplex PCR to sonicate fluid culture applying the same definition as Portillo et al. [116, 117]. The study cohort consisted of 37 patients meeting the definition for PJI. Sonicate fluid culture and multiplex PCR results were discordant in 16 cases (43%); in five cases, *C. acnes* was isolated from sonicate culture but not detected by multiplex PCR—as previously noted, this organism is not detected by the molecular assay used [117]. In 11 cases, organisms were detected by multiplex PCR but not culture; in all cases, the patients had received prior antimicrobial therapy [117].

Overall, 51% of the PJI cohort had prior antimicrobial exposure: in this sub-cohort, sonicate culture was positive in 42% of cases compared to sonicate multiplex PCR which was positive in 100% of cases [117].

As highlighted by both studies, the major limitation of the described molecular approach is that some organisms, such as *C. acnes*, were not included in commercially available kits [116, 117]. Researchers have therefore developed multiplex PCR assay panels specific for pathogens associated with PJI including the panel described by Cazanave and colleagues at the Mayo Clinic, Rochester, Minnesota [118]. Of relevance, this assay panel included primers for organisms such as *Cutibacterium* species and *Corynebacterium* species [118]. This study included 434 lower limb arthroplasty revision cases, including 144 cases that met the modified IDSA criteria for PJI (microbiological criterion was omitted from the definition) [118]. Overall, there were 24 discordant results between sonicate fluid culture and multiplex PCR performed on the sonicate fluid. In four cases, the multiplex PCR was positive with negative sonicate cultures and periprosthetic tissue culture; in these cases, PCR detected *S. aureus*, *Streptococcus agalactiae*, *Streptococcus* species and coagulase-negative staphylococci [118]. In eight cases, culture detected an organism not detected by multiplex PCR including *S. aureus* (five cases), *Candida albicans*, *Capnocytophaga canimorsus* and *Mycobacterium abscessus*. Of note, primers for *C. albicans*, *C. canimorsus* and *M. abscessus* were not included in the assay panel [118]. For organisms that were not detected on the multiplex PCR despite the inclusion of the specific primers in the assay panel, the authors hypothesised that issues with lysis of some staphylococcal isolates may be a potential reason for the failure of the PCR assay to detect these organisms [118]. Overall the reported sensitivities were growth of the same microorganism on two or more tissue cultures 70.1% (95% confidence interval 62.0–77.5%), sonicate culture 72.9% (95% confidence interval 64.9–80.0%) and sonicate fluid PCR 77.1% (95% confidence interval 69.3–83.7%) [118]. Specificity was significantly higher with sonicate culture and PCR compared to tissue culture isolating any organism; however, this difference was not observed when growth of the same microorganism on two or more tissue cultures was examined [118].

In the Proceedings of the International Consensus Meeting on Periprosthetic Joint Infection, PCR was not recommended as a standard diagnostic tool for PJI diagnosis. Instead, it was recommended that molecular methods be reserved for cases of culture negativity [4].

3.9   Histopathology Diagnosis

Histological analysis of periprosthetic tissue is an established adjunctive test for the diagnosis of PJI. An early study by Mirra et al. examined the histopathological features in 34 patients undergoing revision arthroplasty on hip or knee arthroplasties [119]. Features of inflammation, characterised by five or more polymorphonuclear leucocytes per high-power field ($\times500$ magnification), correlated strongly with infection with these changes observed in all of the patients with clinical and/or microbiological findings consistent with infection. These histological features were absent in all patients without clinical and/or microbiological evidence of infection [119]. The diagnostic utility of intraoperative frozen section histopathology has been examined subsequently in a number of studies. A meta-analysis by Tsaras et al. included 26 studies in patients undergoing hip or knee revision arthroplasty [120]. Of note, the cut-off for polymorphonuclear leucocytes per high-power field considered significant varied across the included studies. The authors elected to examine the diagnostic odds ratio and the likelihood ratio as they argued these measures were not dependent on the disease prevalence and were more robust measures of test performance [120]. The pooled diagnostic odds ratio was 54.7 (95% confidence interval 31.2–95.7) with a very strong positive likelihood ratio (12.0; 95% confidence interval 8.4–17.2) and a moderate negative likelihood ratio (0.23; 95% confidence interval 0.15–0.35) [120]. The diagnostic odds ratio did not differ with different polymorphonuclear leucocyte cut-offs [120].

There are a number of limitations with performing frozen histopathology for PJI. Firstly this test requires specialist pathologists familiar with the examination and interpretation of specimen findings, which is not always feasible [1]. In recognition of this issue, the IDSA guidelines instead include the following criterion: "presence of acute inflammation as seen on histopathologic examination of periprosthetic tissue at the time of surgical debridement or prosthesis removal as defined by the attending pathologist" [1]. Secondly, as with other areas of diagnosis, the detection of PJI in shoulder arthroplasties remains challenging. Grosso and colleagues examined the sensitivity and specificity of frozen section histopathology in patients undergoing shoulder revision arthroplasty [11]. The study included 15 patients with aseptic failure, 18 patients with *C. acnes* infection and 12 patients with an infection due to another organism [11]. PJI was based on a combination of preoperative, operative and microbiological findings. The sensitivity for frozen histopathology was lower with *C. acnes* infection compared to other organisms (50% versus 67%, respectively); however, this difference was nonsignificant ($P = 0.15$). The specificity was 100% for both groups [11]. Based on receiver-operator curve analysis, the authors proposed a cut-off of ten polymorphonuclear leucocytes per high-power field be applied, resulting in a sensitivity of 73% for *C. acnes* diagnosis without detriment to the specificity (100%) [11]. Finally, similar to the observations by Bémer et al., the sensitivity of frozen section histopathology differs with biopsy site. In a study by Bori and colleagues, including 69 revision hip arthroplasties, specimens from the femoral stem and acetabular interface membranes had a sensitivity of 83% compared to the pseudocapsule specimens which had a sensitivity of 42% ($P = 0.04$) [121]. The specificity for both specimen types was 98% [121].

3.10   Summary

In summary, there has been increasing research into strategies to optimise the diagnosis of PJI in recent years. Concerted efforts including the publications arising from the International Consensus Meeting on Periprosthetic Joint Infection have provided clarity around diagnostic aspects, such as thresholds for inflammatory and synovial fluid biomarkers to aid diagnosis of PJI. On the horizon, new tests such as α-defensin are being investigated with promising results; however, the wider, external validation of these tests is currently underway which will inform the broader application of these investigations.

In addition to new diagnostic strategies, there has been an increased focus on optimising current culture methods including examination of the optimal methods for specimen collection, processing and culture duration. Furthermore, there is increasing clarity around the optimal application of tests such as sonication and molecular techniques.

References

1. Osmon DR, Berbari EF, Berendt AR, Lew D, Zimmerli W, Steckelberg JM, et al. Diagnosis and management of prosthetic joint infection: clinical practice guidelines by the Infectious Diseases Society of America. Clin Infect Dis. 2013;56(1):e1–e25.
2. Workgroup Convened by the Musculoskeletal Infection Society. New definition for periprosthetic joint infection. J Arthroplast. 2011;26(8):1136–8.
3. Parvizi J, Gehrke T, International Consensus Group on Periprosthetic Joint Infection. Definition of periprosthetic joint infection. J Arthroplast. 2014;29(7):1331.
4. Parvizi J, Gehrke T, Musculoskeletal Infection Society. Proceedings of the international consensus on periprosthetic joint infection. Aug 2013. http: //www.msis-na.org/wp-content/themes/msis-temp/pdf/ism-periprosthetic-joint-information.pdf. Accessed 7 Feb 2017.

5. Alijanipour P, Adeli B, Hansen EN, Chen AF, Parvizi J. Intraoperative purulence is not reliable for diagnosing periprosthetic joint infection. J Arthroplast. 2015;30(8):1403–6.

6. Peel TN, Dylla BL, Hughes JG, Lynch DT, Greenwood-Quaintance KE, Cheng AC, et al. Improved diagnosis of prosthetic joint infection by culturing periprosthetic tissue specimens in blood culture bottles. MBio. 2016;7(1):e01776–15.

7. Zimmerli W, Trampuz A, Ochsner PE. Prosthetic-joint infections. N Engl J Med. 2004;351(16):1645–54.

8. Inman RD, Gallegos KV, Brause BD, Redecha PB, Christian CL. Clinical and microbial features of prosthetic joint infection. Am J Med. 1984;77(1):47–53.

9. Piper KE, Jacobson MJ, Cofield RH, Sperling JW, Sanchez-Sotelo J, Osmon DR, et al. Microbiologic diagnosis of prosthetic shoulder infection by use of implant sonication. J Clin Microbiol. 2009;47(6):1878–84.

10. Shannon SK, Mandrekar J, Gustafson DR, Rucinski SL, Dailey AL, Segner RE, et al. Anaerobic thioglycolate broth culture for recovery of Propionibacterium acnes from shoulder tissue and fluid specimens. J Clin Microbiol. 2013;51(2):731–2.

11. Grosso MJ, Frangiamore SJ, Ricchetti ET, Bauer TW, Iannotti JP. Sensitivity of frozen section histology for identifying Propionibacterium acnes infections in revision shoulder arthroplasty. J Bone Joint Surg Am. 2014;96(6):442–7.

12. Piper KE, Fernandez-Sampedro M, Steckelberg KE, Mandrekar JN, Karau MJ, Steckelberg JM, et al. C-reactive protein, erythrocyte sedimentation rate and orthopedic implant infection. PLoS One. 2010;5(2):e9358.

13. Tsukayama DT, Estrada R, Gustilo RB. Infection after total hip arthroplasty. A study of the treatment of one hundred and six infections. J Bone Joint Surg Am. 1996;78(4):512–23.

14. Peel TN, Cheng AC, Buising KL, Choong PF. Microbiological aetiology, epidemiology, and clinical profile of prosthetic joint infections: are current antibiotic prophylaxis guidelines effective? Antimicrob Agents Chemother. 2012;56(5):2386–91.

15. Barrett L, Atkins B. The clinical presentation of prosthetic joint infection. J Antimicrob Chemother. 2014;69(Suppl 1):i25–7.

16. Parvizi J, Fassihi SC, Enayatollahi MA. Diagnosis of periprosthetic joint infection following hip and knee arthroplasty. Orthop Clin North Am. 2016;47(3):505–15.

17. Kanafani ZA, Sexton DJ, Pien BC, Varkey J, Basmania C, Kaye KS. Postoperative joint infections due to *Propionibacterium* species: a case-control study. Clin Infect Dis. 2009;49(7):1083–5.
18. Dodson CC, Craig EV, Cordasco FA, Dines DM, Dines JS, Dicarlo E, et al. Propionibacterium acnes infection after shoulder arthroplasty: a diagnostic challenge. J Shoulder Elb Surg. 2010;19(2):303–7.
19. Koh CK, Marsh JP, Drinkovic D, Walker CG, Poon PC. Propionibacterium acnes in primary shoulder arthroplasty: rates of colonization, patient risk factors, and efficacy of perioperative prophylaxis. J Shoulder Elb Surg. 2015;25(5):846–52.
20. Levy PY, Fenollar F, Stein A, Borrione F, Cohen E, Lebail B, Raoult D. *Propionibacterium acnes* postoperative shoulder arthritis: an emerging clinical entity. Clin Infect Dis. 2008;46(12):1884–6.
21. Portillo ME, Salvadó M, Alier A, Sorli L, Martínez S, Horcajada JP, Puig L. Prosthesis failure within 2 years of implantation is highly predictive of infection. Clin Orthop Relat Res. 2013;471(11):3672–8.
22. Berbari E, Mabry T, Tsaras G, Spangehl M, Erwin PJ, Murad MH, et al. Inflammatory blood laboratory levels as markers of prosthetic joint infection: a systematic review and meta-analysis. J Bone Joint Surg Am. 2010;92(11):2102–9.
23. Glehr M, Friesenbichler J, Hofmann G, Bernhardt GA, Zacherl M, Avian A, et al. Novel biomarkers to detect infection in revision hip and knee arthroplasties. Clin Orthop Relat Res. 2013;471(8):2621–8.
24. Randau TM, Friedrich MJ, Wimmer MD, Reichert B, Kuberra D, Stoffel-Wagner B, et al. Interleukin-6 in serum and in synovial fluid enhances the differentiation between periprosthetic joint infection and aseptic loosening. PLoS One. 2014;9(2):e89045.
25. Ettinger M, Calliess T, Kielstein JT, Sibai J, Brückner T, Lichtinghagen R, et al. Circulating biomarkers for discrimination between aseptic joint failure, low-grade infection, and high-grade septic failure. Clin Infect Dis. 2015;61(3):332–41.
26. Alijanipour P, Bakhshi H, Parvizi J. Diagnosis of periprosthetic joint infection: the threshold for serological markers. Clin Orthop Relat Res. 2013;471(10):3186–95.
27. Bedair H, Ting N, Jacovides C, Saxena A, Moric M, Parvizi J, Della Valle CJ. The Mark Coventry Award: diagnosis of early postoperative TKA infection using synovial fluid analysis. Clin Orthop Relat Res. 2011;469(1):34–40.

28. Yi PH, Cross MB, Moric M, Sporer SM, Berger RA, Della Valle CJ. The 2013 Frank Stinchfield Award: diagnosis of infection in the early postoperative period after total hip arthroplasty. Clin Orthop Relat Res. 2014;472(2):424–9.

29. Austin MS, Ghanem E, Joshi A, Lindsay A, Parvizi J. A simple, cost-effective screening protocol to rule out periprosthetic infection. J Arthroplast. 2008;23(1):65–8.

30. Schinsky MF, Della Valle CJ, Sporer SM, Paprosky WG. Perioperative testing for joint infection in patients undergoing revision total hip arthroplasty. J Bone Joint Surg Am. 2008;90(9):1869–75. Erratum in: J Bone Joint Surg Am. 2010;92(3):707

31. Tande AJ, Patel R. Prosthetic joint infection. Clin Microbiol Rev. 2014;27(2):302–45.

32. Shih LY, Wu JJ, Yang DJ. Erythrocyte sedimentation rate and C-reactive protein values in patients with total hip arthroplasty. Clin Orthop Relat Res. 1987;225:238–46.

33. Aalto K, Osterman K, Peltola H, Rasanen J. Changes in erythrocyte sedimentation rate and C-reactive protein after total hip arthroplasty. Clin Orthop Relat Res. 1984;184:118–20.

34. Larsson S, Thelander ULF, Friberg S. C-reactive protein (CRP) levels after elective orthopedic surgery. Clin Orthop Relat Res. 1992;275:237–42.

35. Bracken CD, Berbari EF, Hanssen AD, Mabry TM, Osmon DR, Sierra RJ. Systemic inflammatory markers and aspiration cell count may not differentiate bacterial from fungal prosthetic infections. Clin Orthop Relat Res. 2014;472(11):3291–4.

36. Topolski MS, Chin PYK, Sperling JW, Cofield RH. Revision shoulder arthroplasty with positive intraoperative cultures: the value of preoperative studies and intraoperative histology. J Shoulder Elb Surg. 2006;15(4):402–6.

37. American Academy of Orthopedic Surgeons. The diagnosis of periprosthetic joint infections of the hip and knee: guideline and evidence report. Rosemont: AAOS Clinical Practice Guideline Unit; 2010.

38. Bottner F, Wegner A, Winkelmann W, Becker K, Erren M, Götze C. Interleukin-6, procalcitonin and TNF-alpha: markers of peri-prosthetic infection following total joint replacement. J Bone Joint Surg Br. 2007;89(1):94–9.

39. Yuan K, Li WD, Qiang Y, Cui ZM. Comparison of procalcitonin and C-reactive protein for the diagnosis of periprosthetic joint infection before revision total hip arthroplasty. Surg Infect. 2015;16(2):146–50.

40. Liu D, Su L, Han G, Yan P, Xie L. Prognostic value of procalcitonin in adult patients with sepsis: a systematic review and meta-analysis. PLoS One. 2015;10(6):e0129450.
41. Wirtz DC, Heller KD, Miltner O, Zilkens KW, Wolff JM. Interleukin-6: a potential inflammatory marker after total joint replacement. Int Orthop. 2000;24(4):194–6.
42. Shah K, Mohammed A, Patil S, McFadyen A, Meek RMD. Circulating cytokines after hip and knee arthroplasty: a preliminary study. Clin Orthop Relat Res. 2009;467:946–51.
43. Cipriano CA, Brown NM, Michael AM, Moric M, Sporer SM, Della Valle CJ. Serum and synovial fluid analysis for diagnosing chronic periprosthetic infection in patients with inflammatory arthritis. J Bone Joint Surg Am. 2012;94(7):594–600.
44. Trampuz A, Hanssen AD, Osmon DR, Mandrekar J, Steckelberg JM, Patel R. Synovial fluid leukocyte count and differential for the diagnosis of prosthetic knee infection. Am J Med. 2004;117(8):556–62.
45. Santavirta S, Konttinen YT, Nordström D, Bergroth V, Antti-Poika I, Eskola A. Immune-inflammatory response in infected arthroplasties. Acta Orthop Scand. 1989;60(1):116–8.
46. Yi PH, Cross MB, Moric M, Levine BR, Sporer SM, Paprosky WG, et al. Do serologic and synovial tests help diagnose infection in revision hip arthroplasty with metal-on-metal bearings or corrosion? Clin Orthop Relat Res. 2015;473(2):498–505.
47. Parvizi J, Jacovides C, Antoci V, Ghanem E. Diagnosis of periprosthetic joint infection: the utility of a simple yet unappreciated enzyme. J Bone Joint Surg Am. 2011;93(24):2242–8.
48. Wetters NG, Berend KR, Lombardi AV, Morris MJ, Tucker TL, Della Valle CJ. Leukocyte esterase reagent strips for the rapid diagnosis of periprosthetic joint infection. J Arthroplast. 2012;27(8 Suppl):8–11.
49. Shafafy R, McClatchie W, Chettiar K, Gill K, Hargrove R, Sturridge S, Guyot A. Use of leucocyte esterase reagent strips in the diagnosis or exclusion of prosthetic joint infection. Bone Joint J. 2015;97-B(9):1232–6.
50. De Vecchi E, Villa F, Bortolin M, Toscano M, Tacchini L, Romanò CL, Drago L. Leucocyte esterase, glucose and C-reactive protein in the diagnosis of prosthetic joint infections: a prospective study. Clin Microbiol Infect. 2016;22(6):555–60.
51. Deirmengian C, Kardos K, Kilmartin P, Cameron A, Schiller K, Booth RE Jr, Parvizi J. The alpha-defensin test for peripros-

thetic joint infection outperforms the leukocyte esterase test strip. Clin Orthop Relat Res. 2015;473(1):198–203.

52. Colvin OC, Kransdorf MJ, Roberts CC, Chivers FS, Lorans R, Beauchamp CP, Schwartz AJ. Leukocyte esterase analysis in the diagnosis of joint infection: can we make a diagnosis using a simple urine dipstick? Skelet Radiol. 2015;44(5):673–7.

53. Nelson GN, Paxton ES, Narzikul A, Williams G, Lazarus MD, Abboud JA. Leukocyte esterase in the diagnosis of shoulder periprosthetic joint infection. J Shoulder Elb Surg. 2015;24(9):1421–6.

54. Deirmengian C, Kardos K, Kilmartin P, Cameron A, Schiller K, Parvizi J. Diagnosing periprosthetic joint infection: has the era of the biomarker arrived? Clin Orthop Relat Res. 2014;472(11):3254–62.

55. Parvizi J, McKenzie JC, Cashman JP. Diagnosis of periprosthetic joint infection using synovial C-reactive protein. J Arthroplast. 2012;27(8 Suppl):12–6.

56. Tetreault MW, Wetters NG, Moric M, Gross CE, Della Valle CJ. Is synovial C-reactive protein a useful marker for periprosthetic joint infection? Clin Orthop Relat Res. 2014;472(12):3997–4003.

57. Omar M, Ettinger M, Reichling M, Petri M, Guenther D, Gehrke T, et al. Synovial C-reactive protein as a marker for chronic periprosthetic infection in total hip arthroplasty. Bone Joint J. 2015;97-B(2):173–6.

58. Bonanzinga T, Zahar A, Dütsch M, Lausmann C, Kendoff D, Gehrke T. How reliable is the alpha-defensin immunoassay test for diagnosing periprosthetic joint infection? A prospective study. Clin Orthop Relat Res. 2017;475(2):208–15.

59. Deirmengian C, Kardos K, Kilmartin P, Cameron A, Schiller K, Parvizi J. Combined measurement of synovial fluid alpha-defensin and C-reactive protein levels: highly accurate for diagnosing periprosthetic joint infection. J Bone Joint Surg Am. 2014;96(17):1439–45.

60. Frangiamore SJ, Gajewski ND, Saleh A, Farias-Kovac M, Barsoum WK, Higuera CA. α-defensin accuracy to diagnose periprosthetic joint infection-best available test? J Arthroplast. 2016;31(2):456–60.

61. Bingham J, Clarke H, Spangehl M, Schwartz A, Beauchamp C, Goldberg B. The alpha defensin-1 biomarker assay can be used to evaluate the potentially infected total joint arthroplasty. Clin Orthop Relat Res. 2014;472(12):4006–9.

62. Kasparek MF, Kasparek M, Boettner F, Faschingbauer M, Hahne J, Dominkus M. Intraoperative diagnosis of periprosthetic joint infection using a novel alpha-defensin lateral flow assay. J Arthroplast. 2016;31(12):2871–4.

63. Sigmund IK, Holinka J, Gamper J, Staats K, Böhler C, Kubista B, Windhager R. Qualitative α-defensin test (Synovasure) for the diagnosis of periprosthetic infection in revision total joint arthroplasty. Bone Joint J. 2017;99-B(1):66–72.

64. Frangiamore SJ, Saleh A, Grosso MJ, Kovac MF, Higuera CA, Iannotti JP, Ricchetti ET. Alpha-defensin as a predictor of periprosthetic shoulder infection. J Shoulder Elb Surg. 2015;24(7):1021–7.

65. Parvizi J, Jacovides C, Adeli B, Jung KA, Hozack WJ. Mark B. Coventry Award: synovial C-reactive protein: a prospective evaluation of a molecular marker for periprosthetic knee joint infection. Clin Orthop Relat Res. 2012;470(1):54–60.

66. Aggarwal VK, Tischler E, Ghanem E, Parvizi J. Leukocyte esterase from synovial fluid aspirate: a technical note. J Arthroplast. 2013;28(1):193–5.

67. Tischler EH, Plummer DR, Chen AF, Della Valle CJ, Parvizi J. Leukocyte esterase: metal-on-metal failure and periprosthetic joint infection. J Arthroplast. 2016;31(10):2260–3.

68. Deirmengian C, Hallab N, Tarabishy A, Della Valle C, Jacobs JJ, Lonner J, Booth RE Jr. Synovial fluid biomarkers for periprosthetic infection. Clin Orthop Relat Res. 2010;468(8):2017–23.

69. Yeh ET. A new perspective on the biology of C-reactive protein. Circ Res. 2005;97(7):609–11.

70. Deirmengian CA, Citrano PA, Gulati S, Kazarian ER, Stave JW, Kardos KW. The C-reactive protein may not detect infections caused by less-virulent organisms. J Arthroplast. 2016;31(9 Suppl):152–5.

71. Ganz T. Defensins: antimicrobial peptides of innate immunity. Nat Rev Immunol. 2003;3(9):710–20.

72. Shahi A, Parvizi J, Kazarian GS, Higuera C, Frangiamore S, Bingham J, et al. The alpha-defensin test for periprosthetic joint infections is not affected by prior antibiotic administration. Clin Orthop Relat Res. 2016;474(7):1610–5.

73. Deirmengian C, Kardos K, Kilmartin P, Gulati S, Citrano P, Booth RE Jr. The alpha-defensin test for periprosthetic joint infection responds to a wide spectrum of organisms. Clin Orthop Relat Res. 2015;473(7):2229–35.

74. Frangiamore SJ, Saleh A, Kovac MF, Grosso MJ, Zhang X, Bauer TW, et al. Synovial fluid interleukin-6 as a predictor of periprosthetic shoulder infection. J Bone Joint Surg Am. 2015;97(1):63–70.

75. Wyatt MC, Beswick AD, Kunutsor SK, Wilson MJ, Whitehouse MR, Blom AW. The alpha-defensin immunoassay and leukocyte esterase colorimetric strip test for the diagnosis of periprosthetic infection: a systematic review and meta-analysis. J Bone Joint Surg Am. 2016;98(12):992–1000.

76. Cyteval C, Hamm V, Sarrabere MP, Lopez FM, Maury P, Taourel P. Painful infection at the site of hip prosthesis: CT imaging. Radiology. 2002;224(2):477–83.

77. Duff GP, Lachiewicz PF, Kelley SS. Aspiration of the knee joint before revision arthroplasty. Clin Orthop Relat Res. 1996;331:132–9.

78. Miller TT. Imaging of knee arthroplasty. Eur J Radiol. 2005;54(2):164–77.

79. Palestro CJ, Love C, Miller TT. Infection and musculoskeletal conditions: imaging of musculoskeletal infections. Best Pract Res Clin Rheumatol. 2006;20(6):1197–218.

80. Smith SL, Wastie ML, Forster I. Radionuclide bone scintigraphy in the detection of significant complications after total knee joint replacement. Clin Radiol. 2001;56(3):221–4.

81. Delank KS, Schmidt M, Michael JWP, Dietlein M, Schicha H, Eysel P. The implications of 18F-FDG PET for the diagnosis of endoprosthetic loosening and infection in hip and knee arthroplasty: results from a prospective, blinded study. BMC Musculoskelet Disord. 2006;7:20.

82. Zoccali C, Teori G, Salducca N. The role of FDG-PET in distinguishing between septic and aseptic loosening in hip prosthesis: a review of literature. Int Orthop. 2009;33(1):1–5.

83. Kwee TC, Kwee RM, Alavi A. FDG-PET for diagnosing prosthetic joint infection: systematic review and metaanalysis. Eur J Nucl Med Mol Imaging. 2008;35(11):2122–32.

84. Love C, Tomas MB, Marwin SE, Pugliese PV, Palestro CJ. Role of nuclear medicine in diagnosis of the infected joint replacement. Radiographics. 2001;21(5):1229–38.

85. Qu X, Zhai Z, Wu C, Jin F, Li H, Wang L, et al. Preoperative aspiration culture for preoperative diagnosis of infection in total hip or knee arthroplasty. J Clin Microbiol. 2013;51(11):3830–4.

86. Hughes JG, Vetter EA, Patel R, Schleck CD, Harmsen S, Turgeant LT, Cockerill FR 3rd. Culture with BACTEC Peds Plus/F bottle compared with conventional methods for detection of bacteria in synovial fluid. J Clin Microbiol. 2001;39(12):4468–71.
87. Font-Vizcarra L, Garcia S, Martinez-Pastor JC, Sierra JM, Soriano A. Blood culture flasks for culturing synovial fluid in prosthetic joint infections. Clin Orthop Relat Res. 2010;468(8):2238–43.
88. Fink B, Makowiak C, Fuerst M, Berger I, Schäfer P, Frommelt L. The value of synovial biopsy, joint aspiration and C-reactive protein in the diagnosis of late peri-prosthetic infection of total knee replacements. J Bone Joint Surg Br. 2008;90(7):874–8.
89. Williams JL, Norman P, Stockley I. The value of hip aspiration versus tissue biopsy in diagnosing infection before exchange hip arthroplasty surgery. J Arthroplast. 2004;19(5):582–6.
90. Tetreault MW, Wetters NG, Aggarwal VK, Moric M, Segreti J, Huddleston JI 3rd, et al. Should draining wounds and sinuses associated with hip and knee arthroplasties be cultured? J Arthroplast. 2013;28(8 Suppl):133–6.
91. Aggarwal VK, Higuera C, Deirmengian G, Parvizi J, Austin MS. Swab cultures are not as effective as tissue cultures for diagnosis of periprosthetic joint infection. Clin Orthop Relat Res. 2013;471(10):3196–203.
92. Bémer P, Léger J, Tandé D, Plouzeau C, Valentin AS, Jolivet-Gougeon A, Centre de Référence des Infections Ostéo-articulaires du Grand Ouest (CRIOGO) Study Team, et al. How many samples and how many culture media to diagnose a prosthetic joint infection: a clinical and microbiological prospective multicenter study. J Clin Microbiol. 2016;54(2):385–91.
93. Atkins BL, Athanasou N, Deeks JJ, Crook DW, Simpson H, Peto TE, et al. Prospective evaluation of criteria for microbiological diagnosis of prosthetic-joint infection at revision arthroplasty. The OSIRIS Collaborative Study Group. J Clin Microbiol. 1998;36(10):2932–9.
94. Marín M, Garcia-Lechuz JM, Alonso P, Villanueva M, Alcalá L, Gimeno M, et al. Role of universal 16S rRNA gene PCR and sequencing in diagnosis of prosthetic joint infection. J Clin Microbiol. 2012;50(3):583–9.
95. Peel TN, Spelman T, Dylla BL, Hughes JG, Greenwood-Quaintance KE, Cheng AC, et al. Optimal periprosthetic tissue specimen number for diagnosis of prosthetic joint infection. J Clin Microbiol. 2016;55(1):234–43.

96. Hughes H, Newnham R, Athanasou N, Atkins B, Bejon P, Bowler I. Microbiological diagnosis of prosthetic joint infections: a prospective evaluation of four bacterial culture media in the routine laboratory. Clin Microbiol Infect. 2011;17(10):1528–30.

97. Harris LG, El-Bouri K, Johnston S, Rees E, Frommelt L, Siemssen N, et al. Rapid identification of staphylococci from prosthetic joint infections using MALDI-TOF mass-spectrometry. Int J Artif Organs. 2010;33(9):568–74.

98. Peel TN, Cole NC, Dylla BL, Patel R. Matrix-assisted laser desorption ionization time of flight mass spectrometry and diagnostic testing for prosthetic joint infection in the clinical microbiology laboratory. Diagn Microbiol Infect Dis. 2015;81(3):163–8.

99. Borens O, Corvec S, Trampuz A. Diagnosis of periprosthetic joint infections. Hip Int. 2012;22(Suppl 8):S9–14.

100. Butler-Wu SM, Burns EM, Pottinger PS, Magaret AS, Rakeman JL, Matsen FA 3rd, Cookson BT. Optimization of periprosthetic culture for diagnosis of Propionibacterium acnes prosthetic joint infection. J Clin Microbiol. 2011;49(7):2490–5.

101. Schäfer P, Fink B, Sandow D, Margull A, Berger I, Frommelt L. Prolonged bacterial culture to identify late periprosthetic joint infection: a promising strategy. Clin Infect Dis. 2008;47(11):1403–9.

102. Minassian AM, Newnham R, Kalimeris E, Bejon P, Atkins BL, Bowler IC. Use of an automated blood culture system (BD BACTEC™) for diagnosis of prosthetic joint infections: easy and fast. BMC Infect Dis. 2014;14:233.

103. Tunney MM, Patrick S, Gorman SP, Nixon JR, Anderson N, Davis RI, et al. Improved detection of infection in hip replacements. J Bone Joint Surg Br. 1998;80(4):568–72.

104. Tunney MM, Patrick S, Curran MD, Ramage G, Hanna D, Nixon JR, et al. Detection of prosthetic hip infection at revision arthroplasty by immunofluorescence microscopy and PCR amplification of the bacterial 16S rRNA gene. J Clin Microbiol. 1999;37(10):3281–90.

105. Trampuz A, Piper KE, Hanssen AD, Osmon DR, Cockerill FR, Steckelberg JM, Patel R. Sonication of explanted prosthetic components in bags for diagnosis of prosthetic joint infection is associated with risk of contamination. J Clin Microbiol. 2006;44(2):628–31.

106. Trampuz A, Piper KE, Jacobson MJ, Hanssen AD, Unni KK, Osmon DR, et al. Sonication of removed hip and knee prostheses for diagnosis of infection. N Engl J Med. 2007;357(7):654–63.

107. Zhai Z, Li H, Qin A, Liu G, Liu X, Wu C, et al. Meta-analysis of sonication fluid samples from prosthetic components for diagnosis of infection after total joint arthroplasty. J Clin Microbiol. 2014;52(5):1730–6.

108. Malekzadeh D, Osmon DR, Lahr BD, Hanssen AD, Berbari EF. Prior use of antimicrobial therapy is a risk factor for culture-negative prosthetic joint infection. Clin Orthop Relat Res. 2010;468(8):2039–45.

109. De Man FHR, Graber P, Luem M, Zimmerli W, Ochsner PE, Sendi P. Broad-range PCR in selected episodes of prosthetic joint infection. Infection. 2009;37(3):292–4.

110. Hoeffel DP, Hinrichs SH, Garvin KL. Molecular diagnostics for the detection of musculoskeletal infection. Clin Orthop Relat Res. 1999;360:37–46.

111. Mariani BD, Martin DS, Levine MJ, Booth RE, Tuan RS. The Coventry Award. Polymerase chain reaction detection of bacterial infection in total knee arthroplasty. Clin Orthop Relat Res. 1996;331:11–22.

112. Moojen DJ, Spijkers SN, Schot CS, Nijhof MW, Vogely HC, Fleer A, et al. Identification of orthopaedic infections using broad-range polymerase chain reaction and reverse line blot hybridization. J Bone Joint Surg Am. 2007;89(6):1298–305.

113. Clarke MT, Roberts CP, Lee PTH, Gray J, Keene GS, Rushton N. Polymerase chain reaction can detect bacterial DNA in aseptically loose total hip arthroplasties. Clin Orthop Relat Res. 2004;427:132–7.

114. Qu X, Zhai Z, Li H, Li H, Liu X, Zhu Z, et al. PCR-based diagnosis of prosthetic joint infection. J Clin Microbiol. 2013;51(8):2742–6.

115. Kobayashi N, Inaba Y, Choe H, Iwamoto N, Ishida T, Yukizawa Y, et al. Rapid and sensitive detection of methicillin-resistant *Staphylococcus* periprosthetic infections using real-time polymerase chain reaction. Diagn Microbiol Infect Dis. 2009;64(2):172–6.

116. Portillo ME, Salvadó M, Sorli L, Alier A, Martínez S, Trampuz A, et al. Multiplex PCR of sonication fluid accurately differentiates between prosthetic joint infection and aseptic failure. J Infect. 2012;65(6):541–8.

117. Achermann Y, Vogt M, Leunig M, Wust J, Trampuz A. Improved diagnosis of periprosthetic joint infection by multiplex PCR of sonication fluid from removed implants. J Clin Microbiol. 2010;48(4):1208–14.

118.Cazanave C, Greenwood-Quaintance KE, Hanssen AD, Karau MJ, Schmidt SM, Gomez Urena EO, et al. Rapid molecular microbiologic diagnosis of prosthetic joint infection. J Clin Microbiol. 2013;51(7):2280–7.
119.Mirra JM, Amstutz HC, Matos M, Gold R. The pathology of the joint tissues and its clinical relevance in prosthesis failure. Clin Orthop Relat Res. 1976;117:221–40.
120.Tsaras G, Maduka-Ezeh A, Inwards CY, Mabry T, Erwin PJ, Murad MH, et al. Utility of intraoperative frozen section histopathology in the diagnosis of periprosthetic joint infection: a systematic review and meta-analysis. J Bone Joint Surg Am. 2012;94(18):1700–11. Review
121.Bori G, Muñoz-Mahamud E, Garcia S, Mallofre C, Gallart X, Bosch J, et al. Interface membrane is the best sample for histological study to diagnose prosthetic joint infection. Mod Pathol. 2011;24(4):579–84.

Chapter 4
Management of Periprosthetic Joint Infection

Jaime Lora-Tamayo and Oscar Murillo

Abbreviations

AUC	Area under the curve
CNS	Coagulase-negative staphylococci
CRP	C-reactive protein
DAIR	Debridement, antibiotics and implant retention
ESBL	Extended-spectrum β-lactamase
ID	Infectious disease (physician)
IDSA	Infectious Diseases Society of America

J. Lora-Tamayo (✉)
Department of Internal Medicine, Hospital Universitario 12 de Octubre, Instituto de Investigación "i+12", Hospital Univ. 12 de Octubre, Servicio de Medicina Interna (Planta 13), Avda. Córdoba s/n., 28041 Madrid, Spain
e-mail: jaime@lora-tamayo.es

O. Murillo
Department of Infectious Diseases, Hospital Universitari de Bellvitge, Institut d'Investigació Biomèdica de Bellvitge (IDIBELL), Universitat de Barcelona, Feixa Llarga s/n. 08907 L'Hospitalet de Llobregat, Barcelona, Spain

© Springer International Publishing AG 2018
T. Peel (ed.), *Prosthetic Joint Infections*,
https://doi.org/10.1007/978-3-319-65250-4_4

MBC   Minimal bactericidal concentration
MBC$_{stat}$ Minimal bactericidal concentration for bacteria in
           a stationary state of growth
MBEC   Minimal biofilm eradication concentration
MBIC   Minimal biofilm inhibitory concentration
MIC   Minimal inhibitory concentration
MRSA   Methicillin-resistant *Staphylococcus aureus*
MSSA   Methicillin-susceptible *Staphylococcus aureus*
PJI   Periprosthetic joint infection
SAT   Suppressive antimicrobial treatment

4.1   Introduction

Periprosthetic joint infections (PJIs) have become a paradigm of extravascular biofilm-associated infection. The presence of inert material, along with the formation of bacterial biofilm, makes it difficult to resolve the infection with antimicrobial treatment alone. Thus, clinicians must provide aggressive treatments, often *combining surgical and medical interventions.*

Unlike other foreign bodies such as intravenous catheters, prosthetic joints are needed in a given anatomical location in order to provide their function. Indeed, maintenance of joint movement by a functional prosthesis is a relevant goal of therapy for PJI [1]. Therefore, many studies of PJI define cure as a composite outcome including both the achievement of *microbiological cure* and the maintenance of *a functional pain-free arthroplasty*, either by retaining or exchanging the prosthesis. Nevertheless, it is not unusual for these two goals to be incompatible, with one often prevailing over the other.

Given this complex scenario, a synergistic and helpful multidisciplinary collaboration between orthopaedist surgeons, infectious disease (ID) physicians and microbiologists is of paramount importance to increase the likelihood of success. Also, the feasibility of the medical treatment, as well as patient preference, may exert a substantial leverage in the decision-making process.

In this chapter, we will try to outline the main characteristics of treatment for PJI, together with different indications based on the twin goals of achieving cure with a good functional outcome.

4.2 General Principles in the Approach to the Patient with PJI

4.2.1 Surgical Options and Indications for Managing PJI

The surgical options for a patient with PJI are as follows:

1. Intention to cure with prosthesis retention
2. Intention to cure with prosthesis removal:

   (a) With implantation of a new prosthesis (in a one-stage or two-stage exchange procedure)
   (b) Without prosthesis replacement (arthrodesis or resection arthroplasty or amputation)

3. Palliative treatment with implant retention and antimicrobial suppressive treatment

The choice of surgical treatment strongly affects the prognosis and chances of successful antimicrobial treatment, so will be considered the basis for discussing the management of PJI (Fig. 4.1). As discussed below, the surgical options are contingent on the clinical presentation of the infection. In this regard, PJIs are classified following a chronologic criteria in *early* (those developed within the first 3 months after surgery), *delayed* (those presenting between months 3 and 24 after surgery) and *late* (more than 24 months after the placement of the arthroplasty) [2].

Other authors prefer to classify PJI according to the pathogenesis of the infection in *early postoperative* (symptoms beginning within the first month after surgery), *late chronic* (infection developing 1 month or more after the

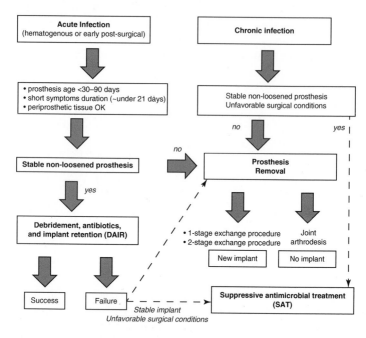

FIGURE 4.1 Algorithm of surgical management of patients with periprosthetic joint infection

placement of the arthroplasty, with an insidious clinical course), *haematogenous* (acute onset at any time after the placement of the prosthesis, in the context of a suspected or documented bacteraemia) and *intraoperative positive cultures* (late chronic infection detected on intraoperative cultures taken at the time of a revision arthroplasty or a one-stage exchange procedure) [3].

Intention to Cure with Prosthesis Retention: Management by Debridement, Antibiotics and Implant Retention Retaining the orthopaedic device, also known as DAIR (debridement, antibiotics and implant retention), is an ambitious option that has several potential advantages:

- Surgical debridement is theoretically a less complex surgery than removing the prosthesis, especially with early postoperative infections where the implant may be soundly fixed. Thus, recovery from this surgery is expected to be easier.

- If successful, DAIR requires fewer surgeries compared with other strategies, such as two-stage exchange procedure, for example.
- Saving the primary arthroplasty allows bone stock to be preserved. This may be important for young patients who still have many years ahead of them and who are expected to need a revision prosthesis in the future.
- Finally, DAIR may also be economically advantageous in some scenarios [4].

While the retention of the foreign body significantly increases the antimicrobial treatment demand, cure rates may be comparable to prosthesis removal if patients are appropriately selected [5, 6]. When DAIR management fails, prosthesis removal is frequently needed, meaning that precious time and resources are lost. Also, compared with patients who undergo prosthesis exchange as the first-line therapy, some reports have suggested that patients have a worse outcome if they require exchange because of a DAIR management failure [7]. Therefore, to maximise the likelihood of success, candidates for DAIR must be chosen with care.

The algorithm for identifying suitable candidates for DAIR, as suggested by Zimmerli et al. [2] and adapted by the Infectious Diseases Society of America (IDSA) [8], is a useful tool for choosing patients with higher odds of benefiting from this strategy [9–11]. According to this algorithm, patients undergoing DAIR should meet the following criteria:

1. The infection must be acute, with a short duration of symptoms. It may be either a haematogenous PJI, with a symptom duration not exceeding 21 days, or an early postoperative PJI, with debridement being performed within 1 month of prosthesis placement.
2. Periprosthetic skin and soft tissues must be in good condition so the prosthesis may be safely covered after surgery.
3. The presence of a sinus tract should discourage from management by DAIR.

4. The prosthesis must be stable and soundly fixed.
5. The infection should be caused by microorganisms susceptible to antibiotics with a good anti-biofilm profile.

While there is wide consensus in the utility of these conditions for considering DAIR management in a given case of PJI, some specific definitions and time limits should be put into context and warrant further consideration (see below The Indication Criteria for DAIR).

Intention to Cure with Prosthesis Removal   The removal of the prosthetic device, in contrast with its retention, facilitates the eradication of the infection by removing the foreign body and necrotic tissue that serve as foci of the infection, thus leading to enhancement of antibiotic efficacy. However, prosthesis removal usually requires complex surgery that may deplete bone stock and reduce joint function.

The attempted eradication of PJI by implant removal and antibiotic therapy may be performed with prosthesis replacement (in a two-stage or one-stage exchange procedure) or without prosthesis replacement (arthrodesis or arthroplasty resection). Prosthesis removal, especially when conducted as a two-stage exchange procedure, is preferred in cases with chronic PJI, and it should be considered an elective strategy in cases of prosthetic loosening, when the surrounding skin and soft tissue are in poor condition and when no antibiotics are available with good activity against biofilm-embedded bacteria. This surgical strategy should also be considered when DAIR has been attempted but has failed, as well as in acute PJI when a DAIR strategy is unsuitable [12, 13].

Palliative Treatment with Prosthesis Retention and Suppressive Antimicrobial Treatment   In some instances, undergoing a curative surgery (either with prosthesis retention or prosthesis removal) may not be acceptable to the patient. This may be for one of several reasons. The patient's condition may be so fragile that the odds of surviving surgery are too low. Also, there might be a clear indication for removing the prosthesis, but without a guarantee of further successful implantation. Else, the results after prosthesis exchange may be expected to be unsatisfactory. The absence of sufficient bone stock and cases where patients have a short life expectancy are good examples of situations where palliation is appropriate. In all these scenarios, the possibility of reducing the symptoms and signs of the infection while keeping a functional (although infected) prosthesis is to be considered.

Long-term suppressive antimicrobial treatment (SAT) is the main palliative option, but does not necessarily preclude performing non-curative surgery, as will be discussed. Actually, in some cases, SAT will be chosen as a salvage option to maintain a functioning arthroplasty when DAIR has failed. Long-term antibiotic therapy may also be prescribed when patients have undergone curative management (prosthesis exchange or DAIR), but where the odds of relapse are perceived as being very high if the antibiotics are withdrawn. This last clinical scenario is rather different, belonging to the ongoing controversy regarding the length of therapy (see below Length of Therapy).

In any case, the decision to use SAT is not straightforward and it deserves careful consideration. Along with the opinion of the orthopaedic surgeon and the ID physician, the patient's personal values and priorities must be considered, because the quality of life with or without prosthesis removal is a subjective and personal issue.

Candidates for SAT must meet the following criteria:

- The prosthesis must be stable and reasonably painless (except if the pain is considered to result from inflammation/infection).
- The microorganisms responsible for the infection must be identified (isolated from reliable samples), so that antimicrobial treatment may be targeted.
- Oral antibiotics with enough activity against the etiological agents of the infection and without long-term toxic effects must be available.
- The patient must be followed up closely, so that any treatment-related toxicity can be rapidly diagnosed, the efficacy of SAT can be monitored and the risks and benefits may be reassessed regularly.

4.2.2   General Principles of Systemic Antimicrobial Therapy for PJI

Antibiotic therapy must be selected taking into account several particularities of foreign body infections, especially (1) the drug diffusion in bone, (2) the presence of bacterial biofilm and a phenotypical bacterial tolerance to antibiotics and (3) the functional abnormalities of phagocytic cells and the presence of intracellular bacteria.

Diffusion in bone is an important factor when considering antibiotic efficacy in the setting of PJI. Bone tissue has a composition with less vascularisation compared with other tissues. The measurement of antimicrobial concentration in the bone is not straightforward, with several techniques used not being standardised. Also, in many studies of uninfected bone samples, there is no information on the ratio of intracellular to extracellular bone or on the free fraction of the antibiotic [14]. Overall, there is some uncertainty on drug concentrations in bone tissue. Bearing these limitations in mind, certain drugs have better concentration in bone, including fluoroquinolones, macrolides and linezolid (serum: bone ratio 0.3–1.2), followed by cephalosporins and glycopeptides (0.15–0.30) and penicillins (0.10–0.30) [14].

The *bacterial biofilm* constitutes a community of microorganisms adhered to a surface that are included within a self-produced polysaccharide matrix. Bacteria within the biofilm exhibit phenotypic changes, which mainly produce the expression of tolerance to antibiotics [15, 16]. Standard antimicrobial susceptibility tests in laboratories, such as the minimal inhibitory concentration (MIC) or the minimal bactericidal concentration (MBC), are performed using planktonic bacteria in a replicating state of growth, which fail to reflect the local environment of bacterial biofilm. These indices have therefore little predictive value of the antimicrobial efficacy against biofilm-embedded bacteria. The performance of adapted in vitro studies has given place to new microbiological indices, such as the minimal biofilm inhibitory concentration (MBIC) and the minimal biofilm eradication concentration (MBEC), which would better reflect the difficulties of antibiotics in a biofilm-associated infection [17]. In addition, previous experimental studies suggest that the use of conventional pharmacodynamic parameters is more appropriate in relation to the stationary-phase MBC (MBC_{stat}), i.e. the area under the curve (AUC)/MBC_{stat} [18]. Overall, improving the evaluation of clinical antibiotic efficacy in this particular scenario is still needed, as well as defining the most appropriate pharmacodynamic parameters that correlate better with the in vivo efficacy.

In any case, the activities of each antimicrobial against biofilm-embedded bacteria are not impaired proportionally. While in some cases the MBIC, MBEC or MBC_{stat} may exceed clinically achievable concentrations, in others these concentrations may be reached by high but non-toxic doses of systemic antimicrobials. For instance, for *Escherichia coli* ATCC 25922, Ceri et al. reported an MIC and MBEC for cefazolin of 1 mg/L and >1024 mg/L, respectively; by contrast, these figures were 0.004 mg/L and 8 mg/L, respectively, for ciprofloxacin [17]. This phenomenon has also been observed in vivo with the tissue cage infection model, where Chuard et al. found that bacteria recovered from the animal's foreign body had MBC values more than 100-fold greater than standard MBC for several antimicrobials [19]. Among staphylococci, susceptibility to β-lactams, glycopeptides and aminoglycosides is significantly altered, whereas fluoroquinolones and rifampin remain more active.

Along with the difficulties in reaching the bone tissue and biofilms, antibiotics may have *impaired diffusion within biofilm structures* and can become trapped in the extracellular matrix. This depends largely on the antibiotic's physical and chemical characteristics and on the presence of extracellular molecules that may impair antibiotic diffusion [16].

In addition, the *intracellular location* of invasive bacteria has also been described in foreign body-associated infection [20, 21], where it acts as a reservoir of infection [22]. Of note, bacteria surviving phagocytosis will neither be affected by the humoral immune system nor be reached by antibiotics that do not possess intracellular activity. Moreover, some antibiotics may penetrate cells, but lack the ability to reach specific intracellular compartments where bacteria hide [22]. As occurs within biofilm structures, intracellular organisms may also enter a quiescent or other adaptive state, such as small colony variants [21–23], which increase their resistance to antibiotics.

Bearing these factors in mind, we can conclude that antibiotics for PJI should have the following properties:

- Good diffusion in bone tissue
- Good diffusion in biofilms
- Good activity against biofilm-embedded bacteria
- Good activity against intracellular bacteria
- A good safety profile that allows long-term administration

4.3   DAIR Management

The true likelihood of achieving cure and retention of prosthetic devices, where the infection is managed by DAIR, is not really known. Many case series have been published, with cure rates reported as low as 18% [24] and as high as 90% in series with very well-selected patients [11, 25]. The success of this complex management strategy depends on several variables. Of these, strict application of the IDSA guidelines and the experience of the surgical team appear to be very important.

Patient's baseline conditions also significantly affect therapeutic outcomes. Chronic renal insufficiency, rheumatoid arthritis, immunosuppressant drug uses and infection of a revision prosthesis are each associated with unfavourable outcomes [26–28]. Clinical presentation is also important, with haematogenous infections (especially in the case of staphylococcal PJI), bacteraemia and high C-reactive protein (CRP) levels associated with worse prognoses [3, 27, 29–31]. Finally, the infectious aetiology and the antibiotic susceptibility profile have a considerable influence on therapeutic outcomes.

In the following sections, we will *discuss* the peculiarities of DAIR management, focusing on key aspects of surgical debridement and antimicrobial therapy based on aetiology of the infection.

4.3.1   The Indication Criteria for DAIR

As mentioned, ensuring that patients meet the IDSA criteria for DAIR can increase the likelihood of treatment success. The rationale for these criteria is to select patients with acceptable local conditions at the joint prosthesis/bone interface, without a chronic infection or mature biofilm and with bacteria that may be treated with antibiotics with a good antibiofilm profile. However, the specific cut-offs and definitions of some of these criteria are somewhat arbitrary, and some observational studies have shown that the violation of these rules does not lead unequivocally to treatment failure.

The definition of what constitutes an acute infection is controversial, because PJI may be considered acute according to two clinical criteria: (a) the duration of symptoms and signs (i.e. time from onset of symptoms to surgical debridement) and (b) the age of the prosthesis (i.e. time from the prosthesis placement to surgical debridement). The first may be difficult to establish because the onset of symptoms can be subtle, especially for postoperative cases when symptoms and signs may be masked by the expected pain and inflammation of the postoperative period. Duration of symptoms is therefore preferred for haematogenous PJI, where the onset is usually more evident.

To this end, a *21-day symptom limit* was established, though it was not based on comparative studies. This cut-off was established on the maximal time that the patients included in Zimmerli's pivotal trial were submitted to debridement [32]. However, it remains unclear whether patients could still have benefited from rifampin plus a fluoroquinolone if they had undergone surgery later. In fact, several studies have addressed this issue and suggested limits other than 21-day symptom duration. For instance, in a cohort of patients with staphylococcal PJI treated mainly with β-lactams, Brandt et al. observed that a debridement delay of more than 2 days was associated with a higher likelihood of failure [33]. However, this time could not be confirmed by later studies using rifampin and fluoroquinolones [27, 31]. Also, in a recent cohort of streptococcal PJI managed by DAIR, a long symptom duration was associated with a poor result, but the 21-day cut-off did not discriminate patients with a better prognosis [34]. Many other case series have also reported that, although a long symptom duration was associated with an unfavourable outcome, no precise and reproducible cut-offs could be provided [24, 35–40].

In this regard, it must be noted that symptom duration may be a surrogate marker of severity. Patients with sepsis, bacteraemia or purulent wound discharge may require surgery earlier than stable patients, yet a short time to debridement would paradoxically be associated with a worse prognosis because of the higher likelihood of failure in this setting [27, 31].

To conclude, no specific time limit has consistently defined a worse prognosis. In this regard, we are certain that candidates for DAIR should be submitted to debridement as early as possible, but we are unable to support the 21-day time limit unreservedly.

By contrast, *the age of the prosthesis* may be a more objective parameter for postoperative infections. Optimal candidates for DAIR are those with an early postoperative PJI, but again the specific definition is not without controversy. Indeed, the concept of early postoperative PJI has evolved over time in several landmark publications, ranging from 1 month [3, 8] to 2 or 3 months [2, 32]. While most physicians will agree that 3 months is a reasonable limit for PJI to be considered as chronic, thereby excluding patients from treatment by DAIR, the debate continues to focus on patients in the timeframe between the first and third month. According to the IDSA guidelines, patients with a prosthesis that is older than 1 month should not receive DAIR, yet a large observational cohort study of staphylococcal PJI showed conflicting results. In that study, the long-term prognosis of patients with a postoperative infection and prostheses aged 1–3 months was similar to that for prostheses aged 1 month or less, whereas patients with a prosthesis older than 3 months had significantly worse prognosis (Fig. 4.2) [27]. These observations were also reproduced in a large cohort of patients with streptococcal PJI [34]. Together, these findings challenge the conventional wisdom that the limit for considering DAIR for postoperative infection should be prosthesis age of 1 month.

In summary, while DAIR should certainly be considered for patients meeting the IDSA criteria, decisions should be made by a multidisciplinary team with expertise in PJI and therapy individualised to the complexities of each patient's condition. On balance, decisions should focus on the stability

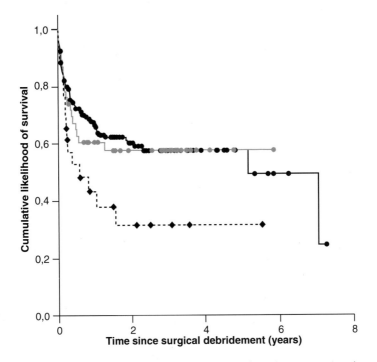

FIGURE 4.2 Survival curves of postoperative (non-haematogenous) cases of staphylococcal periprosthetic joint infection managed by DAIR according to the age of the prosthesis. The figure shows a similar prognosis for 207 cases, with symptoms beginning within the first 30 days after the placement of the prosthesis (*black continuous line*, 38% failures) and 46 patients with onset of symptoms between 31 and 90 days after the index surgery (*grey continuous line*, 41% failures), whereas the outcome of 26 patients whose symptoms began after 90 days was worse (*black discontinuous line*, 62% failures) (long-range test, $P = 0.052$) (Adapted from Lora-Tamayo et al. [27], with permission)

of the prosthesis, the condition of the surrounding soft tissue and the clinical presentation as the most important criteria. In this regard, DAIR should be performed as early as possible and in cases of haematogenous or postoperative PJI with a prosthesis no older than 30–90 days.

4.3.2 Surgical Debridement

The mechanical removal of macroscopic (and microscopic) infection is essential to the success of DAIR management. A suboptimal debridement will probably lead to treatment failure, regardless of the quality of antibiotic treatment and medical management. Therefore, it should be performed by specialist orthopaedic surgeons who are experienced with surgery for infectious complications.

Surgical debridement must be thorough, complete, early and aggressive. It should begin by reopening the previous wound and excising any scar tissue or permanent sutures. All necrotic material, purulent collections and debris must be removed, along with the synovial tissue. Fixation of the prosthesis should be confirmed, and all inert surfaces should be generously irrigated. After this lavage, some authors recommend replacing the surgical field and instruments before wound closure [41].

The replacement of removable components is strongly recommended. This allows not only for the biofilm burden to be reduced but also for greater access to all areas of the joint space. It also facilitates lavage of most component's surfaces. For instance, debridement of the surface of the tibial component of a knee prosthesis cannot be done unless the polyethylene liner is removed, as is valid for the posterior knee compartment (Fig. 4.3). In hip prostheses, it is also recommended that the polyethylene liner and the femoral head be exchanged. Several studies have outlined the benefits of exchanging the removable components of the prosthesis during debridement [41, 42].

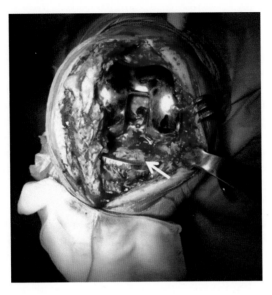

FIGURE 4.3 Surgical debridement of a knee prosthesis. The *arrow* signals debris over the tibial component of the prosthesis, which were not visible until the polyethylene liner was removed

Bearing these factors in mind, most authors recommend debridement to be performed by open arthrotomy rather than arthroscopy. An open wound permits a wider surgical window, an access to remote joint spaces, the exchange of removable components, the excision of infected scar tissues and the repair of damaged tissues. Supporting this approach, a large observational study of more than 100 patients with PJI managed by DAIR showed that debridement by arthroscopy was independently associated with failure (HR 4.2, 95% confidence interval [CI] 1.4–12.5) [26]. Some expert groups have published conflicting data, with good experience in selected patients with infected knee prostheses [43, 44]. In our opinion, the efficacy of arthroscopy for managing PJI needs further evidence before its use can be advocated.

4.3.3   Foreword on Antimicrobial Treatment for DAIR Management

Logically, the recommended antibiotic for a given PJI depends mainly on the microorganisms responsible for the infection and, therefore, on the need for a reliable microbiological diagnosis. The general regimens recommended by the aetiology of the infection may be found in Table 4.1. Before offering further insight into these particular recommendations, we should first consider some generic questions regarding the metabolic status of the bacteria involved in acute PJI and also regarding the total length of therapy.

Planktonic and Stationary State of Growth of Bacteria in Acute PJI   The presence of bacterial biofilm, which involves nongrowing and stationary bacteria, is a major characteristic of PJI and other foreign body infections. Management requires appropriate surgery, and antimicrobials are usually administered in combination and at high doses. In addition, the preferred antibiotic classes can be different to those usually prescribed for common infections where bacteria in the planktonic phase of growth are predominant (i.e. bloodstream infection). In particular, the efficacy of and reliance on β-lactams are significantly reduced in the context of biofilm-associated infection, while rifampin for staphylococci (and maybe for other Gram-positive bacteria, too) and fluoroquinolones for Gram-negative bacilli acquire much greater prominence.

However, acute PJIs, which are usually suitable for DAIR, may also present with a significant component of planktonic bacteria. These infections would be characterised by the presence of bacteraemia, fever, purulent wound discharge, inflammation, high CRP levels and high leukocyte counts. In several large series of PJI with different aetiologies that were managed by DAIR, these parameters were independently associated with the treatment failure, especially in the first weeks after debridement [27–29, 31, 34].

TABLE 4.1 Treatment regimens for patients with periprosthetic joint infection undergoing debridement, antibiotics and implant retention (DAIR)

Bacteria	Time[b]	First-line treatment[d]	Alternative treatment[d]	
Staphylococci	Initially	Daptomycin + cloxacillin	Cloxacillin, daptomycin or vancomycin	
	After	Rifampin + levofloxacin	Rifampin +	Daptomycin or fosfomycin
			Rifampin +	Clindamycin, co-trimoxazole, fusidic acid or linezolid
			Daptomycin +	Cloxacillin, fosfomycin or levofloxacin
			Linezolid	
Streptococci	Initially	Ceftriaxone	Levofloxacin	
	After	Ceftriaxone ± rifampin	Levofloxacin ± rifampin	
		Amoxicillin ± rifampin		

(continued)

TABLE 4.1 (continued)

Bacteria	Time[b]	First-line treatment[d]	Alternative treatment[d]
Enterococci		Ampicillin + ceftriaxone	Vancomycin or teicoplanin; alternatively, daptomycin
		Amoxicillin	Linezolid
Gram-negative bacilli	Initially	β-Lactam[a,c]	Ciprofloxacin or co-trimoxazole
	After	Ciprofloxacin[c]	β-Lactam[a] (consider continuous infusion) ± colistin
			Co-trimoxazole

[a]β-Lactam may be chosen according to the species and common mechanisms of resistance. For *Enterobacteriaceae*, ceftriaxone is a good option; for extended-spectrum β-lactamase or AmpC β-lactamase-producing *Enterobacteriaceae*, ertapenem is the β-lactam of choice; for *P. aeruginosa*, ceftazidime, aztreonam and meropenem are suitable options

[b]Initial treatment refers to treatment immediately after debridement and the first days thereafter (treatment against bacteria in a planktonic state of growth); after refers to targeted anti-biofilm treatment (therapy against biofilm-embedded bacteria)

[c]In infections caused by *P. aeruginosa*, combination of ciprofloxacin with an anti-pseudomonal β-lactam for ≥2 weeks is recommended

[d]Routes and doses, considering normal renal function: ampicillin, 2 g/6 h i.v.; amoxicillin, 1 g/8 h p.o.; ceftriaxone, 2 g/24 h i.v.; cloxacillin, 2 g/4 h i.v.; colistin, 2–4.5 MU/12 h i.v.; co-trimoxazole 800/160 mg/8 h p.o. or i.v; daptomycin, 10 mg/kg/24 h i.v.; fosfomycin, 2 g/6 h i.v; levofloxacin, 750 mg/24 h p.o.; linezolid, 600 mg/12 h p.o.; rifampin, 600 mg/24 h p.o.; teicoplanin, 400–800 mg/24 h i.v.; vancomycin, 1 g/12 h i.v.
For more details, see the text (see DAIR Management)

Also of importance, the possible emergence of antibiotic resistance must be considered. In the setting of acute PJI, this is more likely in the presence of high bacterial inoculum in a high replicative state of growth, such as the days before debridement or just thereafter, when the surgical drains are still present. The risk is also higher for some antibiotic classes such as the fluoroquinolones and rifampin [45].

Thus, in addition to surgical debridement, which is key to reducing the inoculum and fighting the planktonic component of the infection, the initial antimicrobial therapy should include antibiotics with good activity against bacteria in a planktonic state of growth and with a low risk of producing early resistance. In this regard, β-lactams are probably ideal. The likelihood of resistance developing is low, and their ability to clear bacteraemia and replicating bacteria is excellent. Once this initial phase is over, a specific antibiotic regimen may be prescribed that has activity against biofilm-embedded bacteria.

Length of Therapy   Long courses are recommended for PJI managed by DAIR. Current guidelines suggest treatment durations of 3 months (hip prostheses) to 6 months (knee prostheses) [2, 8]. However, many observational studies have shown that such long treatments are probably unnecessary to achieve similar cure rates [46–48]. In this regard, the most robust information exists in the treatment of PJI caused by *S. aureus* and Gram-negative bacilli, using the rifampin-fluoroquinolone combination and the fluoroquinolone monotherapy, respectively. Hypothetically, there may be a time point beyond which extending treatment would not add further benefit. Byren et al. reported a higher risk of failure in the weeks or months after antibiotic withdrawal, but also observed that the risk was not higher for patients treated for shorter periods [26]. Unfortunately, using biological parameters like the CRP does not seem to be a reliable aid when deciding whether to continue or to stop antibiotics [49].

The only clinical trial assessing the comparative efficacy of short and long antibiotic treatment has been recently performed by our multicenter group (REIPI). In this study, 63 patients with acute staphylococcal PJI were managed by DAIR and were randomised to receive levofloxacin plus rifampin during for either 8 weeks (short schedule) or 3–6 months (long schedule). Unfortunately, the study was underpowered, and the non-inferiority hypothesis could only be confirmed in the intention-to-treat analysis, with cure rates of 58% and 73% for the long and short schedules, respectively. There was only a trend toward similarity in the per-protocol analysis (cure rate 95% and 91.7%, respectively) [50].

Overall, we believe that most patients with acute PJI managed by DAIR may be safely treated for 8 weeks with the use of an appropriate anti-biofilm therapy (rifampin-fluoroquinolones for staphylococci and fluoroquinolones for Gram-negative bacilli). Cases with suboptimal debridement or poor resolution of inflammation should be addressed separately.

4.3.4   Treatment Regimens for Staphylococcal Infection Managed by DAIR

Staphylococcus aureus is the most common pathogen associated with acute PJI and so has been the focus of many clinical and experimental studies. According to published case series, the success rate for DAIR management of PJI caused by *S. aureus* ranges from 13% to 90% [6, 25–27, 31, 33, 35, 38]. Our group previously reported a success rate of 55% (95% CI, 50–61%) in a large observational study of 345 patients. Acute infection caused by coagulase-negative staphylococci (CNS) is less frequent, but clinical management appears to be similar [51].

Experimental Research: The Tissue Cage Model   Randomised and prospective studies are very difficult to perform for bone and joint infections. Therefore, much of our knowledge about the activity of antimicrobials in staphylococcal foreign body infections come from the laboratory and animal experiments. In the last years, the tissue cage model, performed with either Wistar rats or guinea pigs, has played a main role to improve our knowledge about the particularities in the pathogenesis of biofilm-related infections [52–54].

The model is considered as a reliable tool to mimic these infections, and it has been widely used to test the activity of antibiotics against biofilm-embedded bacteria [55, 56], providing relevant information for the clinical practice. Indeed, there are other models of device-related infections that have produced very interesting information, such as osteosynthesis-associated osteomyelitis [57] or actual periprosthetic joint infection [58]. However, the tissue cage model has been validated and used by different research groups for more than 30 years, and it has been proven as a reliable easy method that is relatively less expensive.

Briefly, the tissue cage model involves subcutaneously implanting 2–4 perforated polytetrafluoroethylene (Teflon) tissue cages containing two polymethylmethacrylate coverslips. Once the wounds heal (usually 3 weeks later), a standard inoculum is introduced percutaneously (usually 1×10^4 to 8×10^5 colony-forming units). After a variable period (24 h to 3 weeks), which determines the chronicity of the infection, antimicrobial regimens are given during several days (usually 4–14 days). The inflammatory liquid in the tissue cages may then be sampled percutaneously, and viable bacteria measured quantitatively, allowing antibiotic activity to be tested and compared. Thereafter, tissue cages and coverslips may be recovered to perform quantitative counts of any biofilm-embedded bacteria [18, 59, 60]. Table 4.2 summarises the most important studies using this model for staphylococcal foreign body infection [18, 52, 59–81].

TABLE 4.2 Summary of antibiotic activity in the experimental tissue cage model for staphylococcal infection

References	Bact.	Chron/leng[c]	Antibiotics tested	Results and comments
Widmer [18][b]	MRSE	24 h/4 d	DAP, NET, TEI, VAN, CPX, RIF	Experimental evidence of the central role of rifampin-based regimens. RIF + CPX was the best treatment
Lucet [59][a]	MRSA	14 d/7 d	RIF, FLX, VAN	RIF combinations were the most effective therapies
Chuard [52][a]	MRSA	21 d/21 d	RIF, FLX, VAN	
Schaad [61][a]	MRSA MSSA	21 d/7 d	TEI, VAN, RIF	
Schaad [62][a]	MRSA MSSA	21 d/7 d	VAN, IMI, OXA	IMI performed better than OXA for MSSA, but was ineffective for MRSA
Blaser [63][b]	MSSA MRSE	24 h/4 d	RIF, NET, CPX, FLX	Main role of RIF combinations
Cagni [64][a]	MRSA	21 d/7 d	VAN, SPX, TMX, CPX	Evaluation of new fluoroquinolones (not currently available)
Vaudaux [65][a]	MRSA	14 d/7 d	LVX, ALX, VAN	LVX was the most active treatment, with no development of resistance

Vaudaux [66][a]	MSSA	14 d/7 d	DAP, VAN	DAP and VAN activities were alike
Vaudaux [67][a]	MRSA	14 d/7 d	CFB, VAN	DAP performed better than VAN and OXA
Schaad [68][a]	MSSA	21 d/7 d	DAP, VAN, OXA	LVX at high doses proved similar activity as RIF
Murillo [60][a]	MSSA	21 d/7 d	RIF, VAN, LVX (two dosages), LNZ, CLX	Antagonism of RIF + LVX at high doses
Murillo [69][a]	MSSA	21 d/7–14 d	RIF, LVX	VAN and TIG showed similar activity
Murillo [70][a]	MSSA	21 d/7–10 d	RIF, LNZ, CLX	LVX and MXF showed similar activity
Vaudaux [71][a]	MRSA	14 d/7 d	TIG, VAN	DAP at high doses was as effective as RIF
Murillo [72][a]	MSSA	21 d/7 d	LVX, MXF (two dosages)	LVX + RIF and DAP + RIF were the best treatments
Murillo [73][a]	MRSA	3 d/7 d	RIF, DAP, VAN, LNZ	DAP + RIF was the most effective combination
John [74][b]	MRSA	3 d/4 d	RIF, DAP, VAN, LNZ, LVX	
Garrigós [75][a]	MRSA	3 d/7 d	RIF, DAP, VAN, LNZ	

(continued)

TABLE 4.2 (continued)

References	Bact.	Chron/leng[c]	Antibiotics tested	Results and comments
Garrigós [76][a]	MRSA	3 d/7 d	RIF, VAN, TIG	
Garrigós [77][a]	MRSA	3 d/7 d	RIF, CLX, DAP	Anti-MRSA comparative efficacy of DAP + CLX combination
Garrigós [78][a]	MRSA	3 d/7 d	RIF, IMI, FOS, DAP	Remarkable efficacy of DAP + RIF and FOS + RIF combinations
El Haj [79][a]	MSSA	7 d/7 d	RIF, CLX, DAP	Anti-MSSA comparative efficacy of DAP + CLX and CLX + RIF combinations
El Haj [80][a]	MSSA	7 d/7 d	RIF, LVX, DAP	Comparative efficacy of DAP + RIF, LVX + RIF and DAP + LVX
El Haj [81][a]	MRSA MSSA	3 d/7 d	RIF, CLR, DAP	CLR did not prove anti-biofilm effect

Animal employed in the tissue cage model: [a]Wistar rats or [b]Guinea pigs. [c]*Chron* chronicity of infection (time from inoculation to beginning of experimental treatments), *leng* length of experimental treatment, *d* days, *MRSA* methicillin-resistant *Staphylococcus aureus*, *MSSA* methicillin-susceptible *S. aureus*, *MRSE* methicillin-resistant *Staphylococcus epidermidis*. Antibiotics used: *ALX* alatrovafloxacin, *CFB* ceftobiprole, *CLR* clarithromycin, *CLX* cloxacillin, *CPX* ciprofloxacin, *DAP* daptomycin, *FLX* fleroxacin, *FOS* fosfomycin, *IMI* imipenem, *LVX* levofloxacin, *LNZ* linezolid, *MXF* moxifloxacin, *NET* netilmicin, *OXA* oxacillin, *RIF* rifampin, *SPX* sparfloxacin, *TEI* teicoplanin, *TIG* tigecycline, *TMX* temofloxacin, *VAN* vancomycin

Recommended Regimens for Staphylococcal Infection   The initial treatment of methicillin-susceptible *S. aureus* (MSSA) or methicillin-resistant *S. aureus* (MRSA) PJI after debridement should be based on either β-lactams (i.e. cloxacillin or cefazolin) or glycopeptides, respectively [2, 8]. There is a long experience with both antibiotic families for the treatment of staphylococcal planktonic infection, with the likelihood of treatment-emergent resistance being low [45]. However, the activity of cloxacillin may be impaired when the bacterial inoculum is high, and vancomycin's efficacy is often suboptimal. Interestingly, combination therapy with daptomycin plus a β-lactam has shown synergism for both MSSA and MRSA in both in vitro and in vivo models [82, 83], with evidence of good activity against biofilm-embedded bacteria too [77, 79]. These results would encourage the use of daptomycin plus cloxacillin in the first days or weeks after debridement, although clinical experience is lacking.

After this initial period, a targeted anti-biofilm treatment may be started, which is determined by the addition of rifampin.

Schemes Including Rifampin   The activity of rifampin-based combinations against biofilm-embedded *S. aureus* has been shown in several animal models (Table 4.2). Importantly, rifampin resistance can be avoided by adding a second drug [18, 19, 59, 61, 63]. Widmer et al. reported an 84% success rate in a pilot study of patients with orthopaedic hardware-associated infection managed by implant retention and rifampin-based combination therapy [84]. In a similar study of ofloxacin plus rifampin, Drancourt et al. reported an overall cure rate of 74% and a cure rate of 57% among patients managed with implant retention [85].

In the context of this background, Zimmerli et al. published a landmark double-blind randomised clinical trial in 1998, comparing ciprofloxacin alone with ciprofloxacin plus rifampin for orthopaedic hardware-associated acute infection caused by MSSA managed by implant retention. The per-protocol analysis showed a significantly higher success rate for the combined therapy (100% (12/12) vs. 58% (7/12),

$P = 0.02$). This pivotal study forms the clinical basis for using rifampin in staphylococcal PJI managed by DAIR [32].

Later observational studies have confirmed the benefits of rifampin. In a large study of staphylococcal PJI, Senneville et al. observed that fluoroquinolone plus rifampin was independently associated with a lower likelihood of failure (odds ratio 0.40, 95% CI 0.17–0.97) [6]. The benefits of rifampin also seem to apply to MRSA, as shown in experimental models [19, 59, 62, 74, 75]. Case series of staphylococcal PJI where the use of rifampin-based combination therapy was widespread have shown a similar prognosis for MRSA and MSSA episodes [27, 51].

The recommended dose of rifampin is another matter of controversy. In the landmark trial by Zimmerli et al., the dose was 450 mg twice daily [32]; by contrast, the IDSA guidelines use a wider dose range of 300–450 mg twice daily [8]. Other groups have also reported their experience with a dose of 600 mg once daily, similar to the regimen used for tuberculosis. In this regard, the area under the curve (AUC) in relation to the MIC seems to be the best pharmacokinetic/pharmacodynamic parameter for predicting efficacy [86]. It must be noted that the transport of rifampin in the liver is saturable, producing non-linear increases in the AUC for single doses exceeding 300–450 mg. Given this, it is likely that a single fasting dose of 600 mg causes AUCs similar to those seen for 450 mg twice daily [87, 88]. In addition, rifampin dose higher than 600 mg has not been associated with any improvements in outcome [89].

As mentioned, resistance to rifampin develops rapidly and predictably when administered alone, therefore necessitating the use of combination therapy. Beyond this, there is interest in evaluating the relative activities of specific combinations. In this regard, fluoroquinolones have a good antistaphylococcal activity, bone diffusion and bioavailability [14, 90]. Clinical comparison of fluoroquinolone-rifampin regimens with other rifampin-based combinations is scarce, mainly because of the inherent limitations of retrospective studies. Still, there is some indirect clinical data suggesting that fluoroquinolone-rifampin combination therapy may be superior to other regimens. In our large study of staphylococcal PJI managed by DAIR, treatment with fluoroquinolones plus rifampin delayed the moment of failure until the antibiotics were stopped, whereas patients treated with other rifampin-based antimicrobial regimens did fail despite continued treatment [27].

Regarding the specific fluoroquinolone choice, there is wide consensus that newer fluoroquinolones such as levofloxacin or moxifloxacin are preferable to ciprofloxacin because of their higher anti-staphylococcal activity and the lower likelihood of resistance developing during treatment [90, 91]. On the basis of several clinical experiences, expert recommendations and our own opinion, the combination of levofloxacin plus rifampin is currently the best choice in this setting [2, 8]. Moxifloxacin has lower MIC values [90, 92], but the experimental animal model has failed to provide evidence of superiority over levofloxacin [72]. Also, the antimicrobial spectrum of moxifloxacin is unnecessarily wide for treating staphylococcal infection (i.e. it also includes anaerobic microorganisms). Finally, there is evidence that moxifloxacin levels may decrease when combined with rifampin [93].

Sometimes fluoroquinolones cannot be administered with rifampin, either because of intolerance or resistance, as is common with MRSA. In this context, rifampin plus high doses of daptomycin (equivalent to 10 mg/kg in humans) has shown to be the most effective regimen in animal models of MRSA infection [58, 75, 77, 78]. John et al. observed similar efficacies for daptomycin plus rifampin and levofloxacin plus rifampin for fluoroquinolone-susceptible MRSA strain [74], whereas El Haj et al. observed a higher activity of the former combination in MSSA infection [80]. Despite these promising results in animal models, an observational multicentre study of 20 patients with staphylococcal PJI managed by DAIR, with daptomycin plus rifampin used as first-line treatment, failed to provide better results compared with a historical cohort treated with alternative rifampin-based combinations (50% vs. 34% failure rate, $P = 0.265$). However, a lower treatment failure rate during treatment was observed among patients treated with daptomycin plus rifampin, suggesting a higher intrinsic activity of this regimen [94].

Other combinations of rifampin may prevent the development of resistance and are attractive as sequential oral treatments due to their good bioavailability. These include combinations with either linezolid [70, 95, 96], *co-trimoxazole* [97], fusidic acid [25, 98, 99] or clindamycin [100]. In an experimental model, combination with tigecycline plus rifampin has been shown to be equivalent to vancomycin plus rifampin [76], but regarding sequential oral therapy with minocycline plus rifampin, there is limited clinical experience [101].

Schemes Without Rifampin   Despite the evident benefits of rifampin, it has several important drawbacks. One challenge is its ability to induce cytochrome p450 activity, thus increasing the rate of elimination of many drugs metabolised by this pathway [102]. Common examples of these are oral anticoagulants, antiepileptic drugs and steroids. It is important to adjust the dosage of these drugs or reconsider the rifampin prescription. Another important consideration with rifampin is tolerance. Gastrointestinal symptoms are common, especially nausea, vomiting, heartburn and epigastric discomfort. Although this may be improved when administered with food, absorbance is impaired by the increase of gastric alkalinity [102]. Stopping the drug for some days and then reintroducing it may help [32]. Other common side effects include the possibility of liver toxicity, skin rash, fever and flu-like syndrome [102].

Given the drawbacks of therapy, withdrawal or inability to take rifampin is not uncommon. In an interesting retrospective study evaluating 154 patients with PJI treated with rifampin plus levofloxacin, Nguyen et al. observed that rifampin-related adverse events were dose related and occurred in 31.2%, with 18.8% needing to discontinue the antibiotic [89].

Therefore, rifampin may not be an option in some cases, either because of intolerance or resistance. In this situation, the best antimicrobial treatment has yet to be defined, and clinical experience is limited. In experimental models, combinations of daptomycin with fosfomycin [78], levofloxacin [100], cloxacillin [77, 79], linezolid [103] or co-trimoxazole [104] have shown promising results. Other alternatives are high-dose monotherapy with levofloxacin [60, 69], moxifloxacin [92] or linezolid [95].

4.3.5   Infection by Gram-Negative Bacilli Managed by DAIR

Treatment with β-lactams seems adequate for the initial treatment of PJI caused by Gram-negative bacilli, while a predominance of bacteria in a planktonic state of growth exists. A third-generation cephalosporin for *Enterobacteriaceae*, ertapenem for extended-spectrum β-lactamase (ESBL) or AmpC β-lactamase-producing microorganisms or an anti-pseudomonal β-lactam for *Pseudomonas aeruginosa* may all be adequate initial treatments.

After this initial stage, prognosis is largely dependent on the use of fluoroquinolones. In a large observational study of 174 cases, the success rate was significantly higher among patients treated with fluoroquinolones (79%) compared with other antibiotics (41%). Interestingly, the benefits of treatment with fluoroquinolones were also observed for fluoroquinolone-susceptible ESBL-producing bacteria [28]. Previous smaller series have also observed good prognoses when using fluoroquinolones [29, 105]. Therefore, treatment with ciprofloxacin (400 mg bid i.v. or 750–1000 mg bid p.o.) is the treatment of choice for PJI caused by fluoroquinolone-susceptible Gram-negative bacilli. In the case of ciprofloxacin-susceptible *P. aeruginosa*, an initial combination of ciprofloxacin with a β-lactam (i.e. ceftazidime) has given good results [106].

By contrast, the prognosis is poor when using DAIR for PJI caused by fluoroquinolone-resistant Gram-negative bacilli. Usual treatment in this setting is monotherapy with β-lactams or co-trimoxazole, but success rates may be as low as 41–47% [28, 29]. Actually, co-trimoxazole has shown a poor performance in experimental models [107]. In spite of this, its use as sequential oral treatment is frequently considered.

To ameliorate the problems with fluoroquinolone-resistant Gram-negative bacilli, experimental research has provided promising results with colistin-based regimens. Colistin uniquely targets deeper layers within biofilm, offering supplementary effects to a second antibiotic [108, 109]. In a tissue cage infection model of ESBL-producing *Escherichia coli*, Corvec et al. reported a 67% cure rate with colistin plus fosfomycin and a 50% cure rate with colistin plus tigecycline, though no monotherapy could achieve cure [110]. The combination of colistin plus carbapenems for biofilm-embedded *P. aeruginosa* has also been explored in an in vitro model, showing synergy and additivity [111]. In addition, Ribera et al. recently reported 34 cases of orthopaedic hardware-related infection caused by multidrug-resistant *P. aeruginosa*, showing a success rate of 73% for patients treated with continuous infusion of β-lactams plus colistin compared with 32% for monotherapy [112]. Finally, fosfomycin-based combinations may be also considered [110], as may tigecycline, but clinical experience is scarce.

4.3.6   Infection by Streptococci Managed by DAIR

Current guidelines recommend the use of β-lactams for streptococcal PJI [8], despite their poor performance against slow-growing or biofilm-embedded bacteria [113]. Although the prognosis of these infections is believed to be good, with success rates over 89% in small observational studies [114–116], other researchers have contested this claim [117, 118]. In this regard, our group has recently analysed a large international cohort including 462 episodes of streptococcal PJI managed by DAIR. The long-term likelihood of infection cure and prosthesis retention was 57% (95% CI, 52–62%), and treatment with β-lactams was confirmed to be an independent predictor of success. Still, the addition of rifampin improved the results, suggesting that this combination could remain useful once the planktonic phase of treatment has passed [34]. Consistent with this, good outcomes were shown in a univariate analysis of 95 episodes of streptococcal PJI that used rifampin-based therapy (including fluoroquinolones plus rifampin) [119].

4.3.7   Infection by Enterococci

Ampicillin is recommended for enterococcal PJI managed by DAIR [2, 8]. As with infectious endocarditis, attempts have been made to use aminoglycosides; however, not only is the efficacy of this combination unproven, but there is also a risk of toxicity [120]. Other reports support the combination therapy of ampicillin plus ceftriaxone [121, 122]. In a large multicenter observational study including 203 patients with enterococcal PJI (93 managed by DAIR), Tornero et al. found a statistically beneficial effect with rifampin-based combinations for patients with acute infection (symptom onset within the first 30 days of prosthesis placement) [123]. Other possible treatments for enterococcal PJI are vancomycin [120], teicoplanin [124, 125] and linezolid [126]. Finally, there are concerns regarding the activity of daptomycin against enterococci, but some successful case reports suggest this antibiotic as an alternative [127].

4.3.8   Other Aetiologies and Culture-Negative PJI

There is scarce clinical experience with other less frequent microorganisms, especially in the setting of DAIR management. Mycobacteria are very uncommon, fast-growing species being able to produce acute PJI, especially *M. fortuitum*. Overall, there is very little experience reported, and the odds of successful DAIR management seem low [128].

Candida spp. are excellent biofilm formers that may cause PJI, particularly after a bacterial infection or long antibiotic course [129]. Antifungal therapy with azoles has limited efficacy against biofilm-embedded fungi, with activity being slightly better for echinocandins or amphotericin [130]. However, the prognosis is very poor when attempting DAIR for candidal infections, with success rates of just 20% [131, 132]. Until more experience is reported, DAIR management should be discouraged in the setting of fungal PJI. Other options such as SAT, or a two-stage exchange procedure, may produce better results.

Finally, no microbiological diagnosis is possible in some cases of PJI, often because of previous antibiotic use [133, 134]. In a retrospective study of 60 patients with culture-negative PJI, Berbari et al. reported a 71% success rate with DAIR management [133]. It is difficult to make any treatment recommendations in this setting. However, common sense would indicate that one should administer antibiotics with a spectrum that includes the pathogens most often involved in acute PJI (i.e. *S. aureus*, streptococci, Gram-negative bacilli) and also consider the likelihood of antimicrobial resistance based on the local epidemiology (i.e. local prevalence of MRSA). In addition, it is advisable to include an agent with the same antimicrobial coverage as that provided before the culture was taken, because the original antimicrobial may have interfered with the laboratory result.

4.4   Cure Attempt by Prosthesis Removal

4.4.1   Two-Stage Exchange Arthroplasty

The Surgical Procedure The two-stage exchange arthroplasty involves two surgeries [2, 13]. In the first surgery, the prosthesis and all foreign materials (including the bone cement) are removed, an exhaustive debridement is performed and an antimicrobial-impregnated cement spacer is placed into the joint space. Then, systemic antimicrobials are administered for about 6 weeks in most cases. An antibiotic-free period is then allowed (ideally no less than 2 weeks), before the second-stage procedure is performed.

In some cases, infection control is not achieved after the first-stage surgery (e.g. persistent wound discharge, inflammatory signs, etc.), usually because of persistence of the initial infection, but sometimes because of superinfection by new microorganisms. In these cases, further surgery with repeated debridement and exchange of the cement spacer should be considered, followed by new antibiotic therapy.

The second surgery involves the implantation of a new prosthesis, but also includes performing tissue biopsies for histopathological and microbiologic analysis to ensure the eradication of infection. While awaiting this definitive confirmation of PJI cure, patients receive prophylactic intravenous antibiotic therapy. This treatment should target the initial infectious aetiology but also a potential superinfection by different microorganisms, particularly those that are usually part of the patient's skin microbiota [135–137]. Thus, wide-spectrum antimicrobials are recommended as prophylaxis in the second-stage surgery.

Two-stage exchange arthroplasty is considered an effective strategy for managing PJI. In a systematic review of 929 patients, the success rate was 89% [138]. The failure rate after new implantation of hip prostheses is 0–10%, but is slightly higher (5–15%) in studies with 5–10-year follow-up data [138, 139]. In the case of knee prostheses, the rates of failure range from 0% to 18% over short follow-up periods and from 9% to 34% over longer follow-up periods [140, 141].

Systemic Antimicrobial Treatment Between First- and Second-Stage Surgery   Antimicrobial therapy complements the two-stage surgical approach. Therapy can be administered locally (using antibiotic-impregnated spacers) or systemically, but it is most common to combine the two strategies.

Systemic antibiotics have traditionally been administered intravenously over 6 weeks, between the first and second surgical steps. Recent studies, though, have questioned the value of such long treatment courses when antibiotic-loaded cement spacers are used, but at present, there is insufficient evidence to recommend not giving systemic antibiotics [142–144]. Instead, shortening the length of systemic antibiotic therapy in the setting of PJI caused by low-virulent microorganisms (i.e. CNS) could be a more reasonable goal for further research.

It is usually recommended that pathogen-directed antimicrobial treatment be given intravenously throughout. However, recent guidelines and some new studies advocate a short intravenous schedule of 1–2 weeks followed by oral therapy for the remainder of the course [8, 145, 146].

The need to use antibiotics active against biofilm-embedded bacteria (i.e. rifampin for staphylococci and fluoroquinolones for Gram-negative bacilli) has not been proven in the setting of two-stage surgery [8]. For example, rifampin was not used in most series reporting high efficacy (≈90%) of this surgical procedure. This suggests that removing the prosthesis and debriding the periprosthetic bone can eradicate the biofilm, making the anti-biofilm effect of antimicrobials less relevant. Nevertheless, these antibiotics may still be considered in cases in which the surgery was suboptimal or where cement fragments or necrotic bone remain. Also, it would be reasonable to administer a rifampin-based regimen in episodes caused by *S. aureus* with a significant inflammatory load.

Antimicrobial-Loaded Spacers The cement spacers used during the two-stage exchange arthroplasty have two goals: they provide a mechanical support for the joint and high local concentration of antimicrobials. For the first of these, spacers aim (1) to occlude the space left after the prosthesis is removed, (2) to preserve the joint position by avoiding muscle contracture or joint shortening and (3) to maintain joint mobility and patient comfort during the time between the first and second surgery [13, 147, 148].

Spacers may be non-articulated (static) or articulated, though both achieve similar eradication rates. They may be handmade in the operating room but some are preformed, with the latter providing a homogeneous distribution of antibiotic that ensures ISO compliance. Different antibiotics have been used alone or in combination. Overall, the maximal elution from the cement occurs during the first 48 h, decreasing thereafter over the next 15–30 days [149–151].

Although the role of local antibiotic therapy is not well defined in eradicating infection, antimicrobial-loaded spacers are widely used in the two-stage exchange arthroplasty. The selection of resistant microorganisms or the persistence of some bacteria (i.e. small-colony-variant phenotypes) has been observed on the surface of spacers [152, 153], which has led to some controversies regarding the use of spacers in infections caused by multidrug-resistant microorganisms or by those which can be more persistent. Until further data is available indicating clear disadvantages, the use of antimicrobial-loaded spacers should be considered a necessary part of two-stage exchange procedures.

Evaluation of Infection Cure at the Time of Second-Stage Surgery   The objective of the two-stage exchange procedure is to eliminate the infection and to place a definitive prosthesis in a sterile surgical site. While no randomised clinical trials have established the best moment for this new implantation, some cohort studies indicate that surgery after an antibiotic-free period of 2–8 weeks is appropriate [12, 154, 155]. However, the optimal time for placing the new prosthesis should mainly be determined by clinical signs, symptoms and laboratory tests. The IDSA guideline recommends assessing the erythrocyte sedimentation rate, CRP and clinical signs [8]. Nevertheless, some changes of these biomarkers may not be attributable to persistent or new infection. Therefore, the context and the specific clinical scenario of a given patient must be evaluated before implanting the second prosthesis.

Research indicates that analysis and microbiological culture of the synovial fluid obtained from a joint aspirate before the second-stage surgery has low sensitivity for predicting persistence of infection [129, 156]. Given this, it seems more appropriate to take intraoperative samples for histopathological analysis and microbiological cultures during the second-stage surgery. Some authors have used Atkin's criteria to interpret culture results obtained during the second surgery, considering them relevant if ≥1 or ≥2 samples yield a microorganism, with the number depending on the microorganism's pathogenicity [156–159]. Patients with positive cultures at implantation who were treated with a new course of antibiotics had similar prognoses as patients with negative cultures at the second-stage surgery [12].

4.4.2   One-Stage Exchange Arthroplasty

In recent years, one-stage exchange procedures have emerged as an attractive possibility, especially for infected hip prostheses [13, 146]. Although performed less often, the usefulness of one-stage exchange has also been shown in some cases of knee PJI [160–162]. This practice involves removing the original implant and any cement present, followed by aggressive debridement and, in the same procedure, implanting a new prosthesis. The use of antimicrobial-loaded cement to fix the new arthroplasty is common.

This procedure may be considered in non-immunosuppressed patients with chronic PJI, with surrounding soft tissues in good condition, and with sufficient bone stock and if low-virulent microorganisms cause the infection and are susceptible to antimicrobials with activity against sessile (biofilm-embedded) bacteria. This strategy may also be considered in some cases of acute PJI when prosthesis removal and later implantation are not expected to be overly complex (i.e. non-cemented hemiarthroplasties in the elderly).

Antibiotic therapy is started after surgery, but there is still marked heterogeneity in the regimens used. The total length of therapy (intravenous plus oral) varies widely from 10 days to 6 months. In the setting of staphylococcal infections, the IDSA guideline recommends using intravenous antibiotics for 2–6 weeks, followed by an oral rifampin-based combination to a total of 3 months of treatment [8]. Some authors have also reported their experience using antibiotics to reduce the bacterial load and the risk of contamination of the new arthroplasty before surgery [163, 164].

Overall, one-stage exchange arthroplasty appears to offer success rates comparable to those with two-stage exchange arthroplasty. However, there have been no randomised trials directly comparing these two strategies. A cure rate of 87% was reported in a recent meta-analysis of 375 patients undergoing one-stage exchange arthroplasty [138, 165]. Despite the heterogeneity of the results included, the cure rates reported suggest that the surgeon's ability is crucial for the success of this strategy, which needs an exhaustive debridement and removal of all foreign bodies and necrotic tissues.

4.4.3   Arthroplasty Resection Without New Implantation (Arthrodesis)

This strategy involves removing the prosthesis without replacing it with a new implant. It is considered when implantation of a new device is not viable because of anatomical restrictions, the patient's baseline condition, or the patient's functional level. Some patients for whom a two-stage exchange arthroplasty was initially planned may end up being considered for a definitive arthrodesis due to adverse or unforeseen clinical events after the first-stage procedure. In these patients, the "temporary" spacer will remain in place in the joint indefinitely.

In a resection arthroplasty of the hip, which is called a Girdlestone procedure, the femoral diaphysis is fixed in the acetabulum [166]. The strategy is typically associated with impairment of function, and patients usually need assistance with ambulation. However, the procedure does allow for a new prosthesis to be implanted later, if deemed appropriate.

Knee arthrodesis can be performed by external fixation or by intramedullary nailing [167, 168] and usually does not prevent patients from mobilising. In highly complex surgical scenarios, or when patients have a short life expectancy, placing a permanent cement spacer may be considered [169].

Lastly, in some exceptional cases, amputation may be necessary.

Antimicrobial treatment used following arthrodesis is similar to that used with the two-stage exchange procedure; thus, most common regimens involve giving antibiotics for 4–6 weeks.

4.5   Palliative Treatment: SAT

This therapeutic option is not an infrequent choice, especially for elderly patients [170, 171]. As previously mentioned, the goal of this approach is to retain a functioning arthroplasty, with a minimum signs and symptoms of infection (i.e. a pain-free prosthesis with no productive sinus tracts).

However, the success of SAT has been poorly measured in the literature, probably because of the subjectivity of the endpoints and an underreporting of cases with unfavourable outcome. This is especially so for patients who are finally submitted to salvage therapy with prosthesis removal and who are therefore not counted as having been managed by SAT. Clinical research is also mainly retrospective, with end-points often differing across studies (e.g. avoidance of surgery or repression of symptoms). Bearing these limitations in mind, success rates are reported to range from as low as 23% to as high as 84% [92, 170–173].

Despite not being done with curative intent, some authors have described performing surgical debridement before SAT [172, 173]. This management offers the advantage of reducing the infectious inoculum, thereby theoretically increasing the chances that SAT will be successful, and allows reliable samples to be obtained so that the responsible microorganism is correctly identified. Otherwise, a joint aspirate may be indicated to help diagnose the aetiology and choose a targeted sustainable antimicrobial therapy.

As previously mentioned, antibiotics should be active against microorganisms involved and should also be non-toxic in the long term. Most case series have reported that minocycline plus rifampin, or β-lactams alone, can be used for this purpose [170–172].

4.6   Conclusions

The management of PJI remains a challenging issue, requiring a combined therapy of surgery and antimicrobial treatment, which should be designed by a multidisciplinary team with expertise in the field, including orthopaedic surgeons, ID physicians and microbiologists. The possibilities of curing infection must be weighed against the risks of surgery and the odds of success. The treatment decision follows three main pathways: cure by implant retention, cure by prosthesis removal or palliation with implant retention. The aetiology, the patient's baseline condition and the IDSA criteria for DAIR are useful tools that can help with this decision process. In any of these scenarios, however, a sophisticated antimicrobial therapy must be designed. Treatment should never be made more difficult than it needs to be by failing to obtain a microbiological diagnosis, emphasising the need for reliable cultures.

Attempts to achieve cure with implant retention requires a thorough and prompt debridement, ideally including the exchange of removable components. Retention of the foreign body necessitates a demanding antimicrobial treatment in which the use of rifampin, for staphylococci, and fluoroquinolones, for Gram-negative microorganisms, is of paramount importance.

Prosthesis removal, which is usually reserved for chronic infections, requires a more complex surgical management. However, it does allow for the removal of the foreign body and the attached biofilm, thereby theoretically decreasing the complexity of antimicrobial treatment. Two-stage exchange procedure is considered the treatment of choice in this situation. However, the performance and reported success rate of one-stage exchange arthroplasty is increasing in the last years. Currently, the choice between one- and two-stage procedures depends on the experience of the surgeons, the aetiology of the infection, the location of the prosthesis and the condition of the periprosthetic skin and soft tissues. In the setting of a two-stage exchange procedure, local antibiotics carried by the cement spacer may provide high concentrations of the drug, which would not be possible by systemic therapy alone. Confirmation of infection eradication at the time of implantation for two-stage exchange procedures is an important issue that may require the prescription of new courses of antibiotics.

Finally, performing complex surgery is not always possible or desirable. In these cases, the use of prolonged suppressive antibiotic therapy that can alleviate the patient's infection while retaining a functioning arthroplasty should be considered.

Acknowledgments We thank Michael Maudsley (Universidad de Barcelona) for reviewing the English manuscript. J. L-T is supported by a clinical research contract "Sara Borrell" (Instituto de Salud Carlos III, Ministerio de Economía y Competitividad, CD14/00176).

References

1. Cobo J, Del Pozo JL. Prosthetic joint infection: diagnosis and management. Expert Rev Anti-Infect Ther. 2011;9(9):787–802.
2. Zimmerli W, Trampuz A, Ochsner PE. Prosthetic-joint infections. New Engl J Med. 2004;351(16):1645–54.
3. Tsukayama DT, Estrada R, Gustilo RB. Infection after total hip arthroplasty. A study of the treatment of one hundred and six infections. J Bone Joint Surg Am. 1996;78(4):512–23.
4. Fisman DN, Reilly DT, Karchmer AW, Goldie SJ. Clinical effectiveness and cost-effectiveness of 2 management strategies for infected total hip arthroplasty in the elderly. Clin Infect Dis. 2001;32(3):419–30.
5. Achermann Y, Stasch P, Preiss S, Lucke K, Vogt M. Characteristics and treatment outcomes of 69 cases with early prosthetic joint infections of the hip and knee. Infection. 2014;42(3):511–9.
6. Senneville E, Joulie D, Legout L, Valette M, Dezeque H, Beltrand E, et al. Outcome and predictors of treatment failure in total hip/knee prosthetic joint infections due to Staphylococcus aureus. Clin Infect Dis. 2011;53(4):334–40.
7. Sherrell JC, Fehring TK, Odum S, Hansen E, Zmistowski B, Dennos A, et al. The Chitranjan Ranawat Award: fate of two-

stage reimplantation after failed irrigation and debridement for periprosthetic knee infection. Clin Orthop Relat Res. 2011;469(1):18–25.

8. Osmon DR, Berbari EF, Berendt AR, Lew D, Zimmerli W, Steckelberg JM, et al. Diagnosis and management of prosthetic joint infection: clinical practice guidelines by the Infectious Diseases Society of America. Clin Infect Dis. 2013;56(1):e1–e25.

9. Laffer RR, Graber P, Ochsner PE, Zimmerli W. Outcome of prosthetic knee-associated infection: evaluation of 40 consecutive episodes at a single centre. Clin Microbiol Infect. 2006;12(5):433–9.

10. Sendi P, Christensson B, Uckay I, Trampuz A, Achermann Y, Boggian K, et al. Group B streptococcus in prosthetic hip and knee joint-associated infections. J Hosp Infect. 2011;79(1):64–9.

11. Tschudin-Sutter S, Frei R, Dangel M, Jakob M, Balmelli C, Schaefer DJ, et al. Validation of a treatment algorithm for orthopaedic implant-related infections with device-retention-results from a prospective observational cohort study. Clin Microbiol Infect. 2016;22(5):457.e1–9.

12. Bejon P, Berendt A, Atkins BL, Green N, Parry H, Masters S, et al. Two-stage revision for prosthetic joint infection: predictors of outcome and the role of reimplantation microbiology. J Antimicrob Chemother. 2010;65(3):569–75.

13. Tande AJ, Patel R. Prosthetic joint infection. Clin Microbiol Rev. 2014;27(2):302–45.

14. Landersdorfer CB, Bulitta JB, Kinzig M, Holzgrabe U, Sorgel F. Penetration of antibacterials into bone: pharmacokinetic, pharmacodynamic and bioanalytical considerations. Clin Pharmacokinet. 2009;48(2):89–124.

15. Costerton JW, Stewart PS, Greenberg EP. Bacterial biofilms: a common cause of persistent infections. Science. 1999;284(5418):1318–22.

16. Stewart PS, Costerton JW. Antibiotic resistance of bacteria in biofilms. Lancet. 2001;358(9276):135–8.

17. Ceri H, Olson ME, Stremick C, Read RR, Morck D, Buret A. The Calgary Biofilm Device: new technology for rapid determination of antibiotic susceptibilities of bacterial biofilms. J Clin Microbiol. 1999;37(6):1771–6.

18. Widmer AF, Frei R, Rajacic Z, Zimmerli W. Correlation between in vivo and in vitro efficacy of antimicrobial agents against foreign body infections. J Infect Dis. 1990;162(1):96–102.

19. Chuard C, Herrmann M, Vaudaux P, Waldvogel FA, Lew DP. Successful therapy of experimental chronic foreign-body infection due to methicillin-resistant Staphylococcus aureus by

antimicrobial combinations. Antimicrob Agents Chemother. 1991;35(12):2611–6.

20. Murillo O, Pachon ME, Euba G, Verdaguer R, Carreras M, Cabellos C, et al. Intracellular antimicrobial activity appearing as a relevant factor in antibiotic efficacy against an experimental foreign-body infection caused by Staphylococcus aureus. J Antimicrob Chemother. 2009;64(5):1062–6.

21. Sendi P, Rohrbach M, Graber P, Frei R, Ochsner PE, Zimmerli W. Staphylococcus aureus small colony variants in prosthetic joint infection. Clin Infect Dis. 2006;43(8):961–7.

22. Maurin M, Raoult D. Intracellular organisms. Int J Antimicrob Agents. 1997;9(1):61–70.

23. Proctor RA, Peters G. Small colony variants in staphylococcal infections: diagnostic and therapeutic implications. Clin Infect Dis. 1998;27(3):419–22.

24. Burger RR, Basch T, Hopson CN. Implant salvage in infected total knee arthroplasty. Clin Orthop Relat Res. 1991;273:105–12.

25. Aboltins CA, Page MA, Buising KL, Jenney AW, Daffy JR, Choong PF, et al. Treatment of staphylococcal prosthetic joint infections with debridement, prosthesis retention and oral rifampicin and fusidic acid. Clin Microbiol Infect. 2007;13(6):586–91.

26. Byren I, Bejon P, Atkins BL, Angus B, Masters S, McLardy-Smith P, et al. One hundred and twelve infected arthroplasties treated with 'DAIR' (debridement, antibiotics and implant retention): antibiotic duration and outcome. J Antimicrob Chemother. 2009;63(6):1264–71.

27. Lora-Tamayo J, Murillo O, Iribarren JA, Soriano A, Sanchez-Somolinos M, Baraia-Etxaburu JM, et al. A large multi-center study of methicillin-susceptible and methicillin-resistant Staphylococcus aureus prosthetic joint infections managed with implant retention. Clin Infect Dis. 2013;56(2):182–94.

28. Rodriguez-Pardo D, Pigrau C, Lora-Tamayo J, Soriano A, del Toro MD, Cobo J, et al. Gram-negative prosthetic joint infection: outcome of a debridement, antibiotics and implant retention approach. A large multicentre study. Clin Microbiol Infect. 2014;20(11):O911–9.

29. Martinez-Pastor JC, Munoz-Mahamud E, Vilchez F, Garcia-Ramiro S, Bori G, Sierra J, et al. Outcome of acute prosthetic joint infections due to gram-negative bacilli treated with open debridement and retention of the prosthesis. Antimicrob Agents Chemother. 2009;53(11):4772–7.

30. Sendi P, Banderet F, Graber P, Zimmerli W. Clinical comparison between exogenous and haematogenous periprosthetic joint infections caused by Staphylococcus aureus. Clin Microbiol Infect. 2011;17(7):1098–100.

31. Vilchez F, Martinez-Pastor JC, Garcia-Ramiro S, Bori G, Macule F, Sierra J, et al. Outcome and predictors of treatment failure in early post-surgical prosthetic joint infections due to Staphylococcus aureus treated with debridement. Clin Microbiol Infect. 2011;17(3):439–44.

32. Zimmerli W, Widmer AF, Blatter M, Frei R, Ochsner PE. Role of rifampin for treatment of orthopedic implant-related staphylococcal infections: a randomized controlled trial. Foreign-Body Infection (FBI) Study Group. JAMA. 1998;279(19):1537–41.

33. Brandt CM, Sistrunk WW, Duffy MC, Hanssen AD, Steckelberg JM, Ilstrup DM, et al. Staphylococcus aureus prosthetic joint infection treated with debridement and prosthesis retention. Clin Infect Dis. 1997;24(5):914–9.

34. Lora-Tamayo J, Senneville É, Ribera A, Berard L, Dupon M, Zeller V, et al. The not-so-good prognosis of streptococcal periprosthetic joint infection managed by implant retention: the results of a large multicenter study. Clin Infect Dis. 2017; 64(12): 1742–52.

35. Barberan J, Aguilar L, Carroquino G, Gimenez MJ, Sanchez B, Martinez D, et al. Conservative treatment of staphylococcal prosthetic joint infections in elderly patients. Am J Med. 2006;119(11):993.e7–10.

36. Geurts JA, Janssen DM, Kessels AG, Walenkamp GH. Good results in postoperative and hematogenous deep infections of 89 stable total hip and knee replacements with retention of prosthesis and local antibiotics. Acta Orthop. 2013;84(6):509–16.

37. Hsieh PH, Lee MS, Hsu KY, Chang YH, Shih HN, Ueng SW. Gram-negative prosthetic joint infections: risk factors and outcome of treatment. Clin Infect Dis. 2009;49(7):1036–43.

38. Marculescu CE, Berbari EF, Hanssen AD, Steckelberg JM, Harmsen SW, Mandrekar JN, et al. Outcome of prosthetic joint infections treated with debridement and retention of components. Clin Infect Dis. 2006;42(4):471–8.

39. Schoifet SD, Morrey BF. Treatment of infection after total knee arthroplasty by debridement with retention of the components. J Bone Joint Surg Am. 1990;72(9):1383–90.

40. Tattevin P, Cremieux AC, Pottier P, Huten D, Carbon C. Prosthetic joint infection: when can prosthesis salvage be considered? Clin Infect Dis. 1999;29(2):292–5.

41. Haasper C, Buttaro M, Hozack W, Aboltins CA, Borens O, Callaghan JJ, et al. Irrigation and debridement. J Orthop Res. 2014;32(Suppl 1):S130–5.

42. Choi HR, von Knoch F, Zurakowski D, Nelson SB, Malchau H. Can implant retention be recommended for treatment of infected TKA? Clin Orthop Relat Res. 2011;469(4):961–9.

43. Chung JY, Ha CW, Park YB, Song YJ, Yu KS. Arthroscopic debridement for acutely infected prosthetic knee: any role for infection control and prosthesis salvage? Arthroscopy. 2014;30(5):599–606.

44. Dixon P, Parish EN, Cross MJ. Arthroscopic debridement in the treatment of the infected total knee replacement. J Bone Joint Surg (Br). 2004;86(1):39–42.

45. Sendi P, Zimmerli W. Antimicrobial treatment concepts for orthopaedic device-related infection. Clin Microbiol Infect. 2012;18(12):1176–84.

46. Bernard L, Legout L, Zurcher-Pfund L, Stern R, Rohner P, Peter R, et al. Six weeks of antibiotic treatment is sufficient following surgery for septic arthroplasty. J Infect. 2010;61(2):125–32.

47. Puhto AP, Puhto T, Syrjala H. Short-course antibiotics for prosthetic joint infections treated with prosthesis retention. Clin Microbiol Infect. 2012;18(11):1143–8.

48. Soriano A, Garcia S, Bori G, Almela M, Gallart X, Macule F, et al. Treatment of acute post-surgical infection of joint arthroplasty. Clin Microbiol Infect. 2006;12(9):930–3.

49. Piso RJ, Elke R. Antibiotic treatment can be safely stopped in asymptomatic patients with prosthetic joint infections despite persistent elevated C-reactive protein values. Infection. 2010;38(4):293–6.

50. Lora-Tamayo J, Euba G, Cobo J, Horcajada JP, Soriano A, Sandoval E, et al. Short- versus long-duration levofloxacin plus rifampicin for acute staphylococcal prosthetic joint infection managed with implant retention: a randomised clinical trial. Int J Antimicrob Agents. 2016;48(3):310–6.

51. Tornero E, Morata L, Martinez-Pastor JC, Bori G, Mensa J, Soriano A. Prosthetic joint infections due to methicillin-resistant and methicillin-susceptible staphylococci treated with open debridement and retention of the prosthesis. Rev Esp Quimioter. 2013;26(4):353–9.

52. Chuard C, Lucet JC, Rohner P, Herrmann M, Auckenthaler R, Waldvogel FA, et al. Resistance of Staphylococcus aureus recovered from infected foreign body in vivo to killing by antimicrobials. J Infect Dis. 1991;163(6):1369–73.

53. Zimmerli W, Lew PD, Waldvogel FA. Pathogenesis of foreign body infection. Evidence for a local granulocyte defect. J Clin Invest. 1984;73(4):1191–200.

54. Zimmerli W, Waldvogel FA, Vaudaux P, Nydegger UE. Pathogenesis of foreign body infection: description and characteristics of an animal model. J Infect Dis. 1982;146(4):487–97.

55. Coenye T, Nelis HJ. In vitro and in vivo model systems to study microbial biofilm formation. J Microbiol Methods. 2010;83(2):89–105.

56. Zak O, Sande MA. Handbook of animal models of infection. experimental models in antimicrobial chemotherapy. London: Academic; 1999.

57. Del Pozo JL, Rouse MS, Euba G, Kang CI, Mandrekar JN, Steckelberg JM, et al. The electricidal effect is active in an experimental model of Staphylococcus epidermidis chronic foreign body osteomyelitis. Antimicrob Agents Chemother. 2009;53(10):4064–8.

58. Saleh-Mghir A, Muller-Serieys C, Dinh A, Massias L, Cremieux AC. Adjunctive rifampin is crucial to optimizing daptomycin efficacy against rabbit prosthetic joint infection due to methicillin-resistant Staphylococcus aureus. Antimicrob Agents Chemother. 2011;55(10):4589–93.

59. Lucet JC, Herrmann M, Rohner P, Auckenthaler R, Waldvogel FA, Lew DP. Treatment of experimental foreign body infection caused by methicillin-resistant Staphylococcus aureus. Antimicrob Agents Chemother. 1990;34(12):2312–7.

60. Murillo O, Domenech A, Garcia A, Tubau F, Cabellos C, Gudiol F, et al. Efficacy of high doses of levofloxacin in experimental foreign-body infection by methicillin-susceptible Staphylococcus aureus. Antimicrob Agents Chemother. 2006;50(12):4011–7.

61. Schaad HJ, Chuard C, Vaudaux P, Waldvogel FA, Lew DP. Teicoplanin alone or combined with rifampin compared with vancomycin for prophylaxis and treatment of experimental foreign body infection by methicillin-resistant Staphylococcus aureus. Antimicrob Agents Chemother. 1994;38(8):1703–10.

62. Schaad HJ, Chuard C, Vaudaux P, Rohner P, Waldvogel FA, Lew DP. Comparative efficacies of imipenem, oxacillin and vancomycin for therapy of chronic foreign body infection due

to methicillin-susceptible and -resistant Staphylococcus aureus. J Antimicrob Chemother. 1994;33(6):1191–200.

63. Blaser J, Vergeres P, Widmer AF, Zimmerli W. In vivo verification of in vitro model of antibiotic treatment of device-related infection. Antimicrob Agents Chemother. 1995;39(5):1134–9.

64. Cagni A, Chuard C, Vaudaux PE, Schrenzel J, Lew DP. Comparison of sparfloxacin, temafloxacin, and ciprofloxacin for prophylaxis and treatment of experimental foreign-body infection by methicillin-resistant Staphylococcus aureus. Antimicrob Agents Chemother. 1995;39(8):1655–60.

65. Vaudaux P, Francois P, Bisognano C, Schrenzel J, Lew DP. Comparison of levofloxacin, alatrofloxacin, and vancomycin for prophylaxis and treatment of experimental foreign-body-associated infection by methicillin-resistant Staphylococcus aureus. Antimicrob Agents Chemother. 2002;46(5):1503–9.

66. Vaudaux P, Francois P, Bisognano C, Li D, Lew DP, Schrenzel J. Comparative efficacy of daptomycin and vancomycin in the therapy of experimental foreign body infection due to Staphylococcus aureus. J Antimicrob Chemother. 2003;52(1):89–95.

67. Vaudaux P, Gjinovci A, Bento M, Li D, Schrenzel J, Lew DP. Intensive therapy with ceftobiprole medocaril of experimental foreign-body infection by methicillin-resistant Staphylococcus aureus. Antimicrob Agents Chemother. 2005;49(9):3789–93.

68. Schaad HJ, Bento M, Lew DP, Vaudaux P. Evaluation of high-dose daptomycin for therapy of experimental Staphylococcus aureus foreign body infection. BMC Infect Dis. 2006;6:74.

69. Murillo O, Pachon ME, Euba G, Verdaguer R, Tubau F, Cabellos C, et al. Antagonistic effect of rifampin on the efficacy of high-dose levofloxacin in staphylococcal experimental foreign-body infection. Antimicrob Agents Chemother. 2008;52(10):3681–6.

70. Murillo O, Domenech A, Euba G, Verdaguer R, Tubau F, Cabo J, et al. Efficacy of linezolid alone and in combination with rifampin in staphylococcal experimental foreign-body infection. J Infect. 2008;57(3):229–35.

71. Vaudaux P, Fleury B, Gjinovci A, Huggler E, Tangomo-Bento M, Lew DP. Comparison of tigecycline and vancomycin for treatment of experimental foreign-body infection due to methicillin-resistant Staphylococcus aureus. Antimicrob Agents Chemother. 2009;53(7):3150–2.

72. Murillo O, Pachon ME, Euba G, Verdaguer R, Tubau F, Cabellos C, et al. High doses of levofloxacin vs moxifloxacin against

staphylococcal experimental foreign-body infection: the effect of higher MIC-related pharmacokinetic parameters on efficacy. J Infect. 2009;58(3):220–6.

73. Murillo O, Garrigós C, Pachón ME, Euba G, Verdaguer R, Cabellos C, et al. Efficacy of high doses of daptomycin versus alternative therapies against experimental foreign-body infection by methicillin-resistant Staphylococcus aureus. Antimicrob Agents Chemother. 2009;53(10):4252–7.

74. John AK, Baldoni D, Haschke M, Rentsch K, Schaerli P, Zimmerli W, et al. Efficacy of daptomycin in implant-associated infection due to methicillin-resistant Staphylococcus aureus: importance of combination with rifampin. Antimicrob Agents Chemother. 2009;53(7):2719–24.

75. Garrigos C, Murillo O, Euba G, Verdaguer R, Tubau F, Cabellos C, et al. Efficacy of usual and high doses of daptomycin in combination with rifampin versus alternative therapies in experimental foreign-body infection by methicillin-resistant Staphylococcus aureus. Antimicrob Agents Chemother. 2010;54(12):5251–6.

76. Garrigos C, Murillo O, Euba G, Verdaguer R, Tubau F, Cabellos C, et al. Efficacy of tigecycline alone and with rifampin in foreign-body infection by methicillin-resistant Staphylococcus aureus. J Infect. 2011;63(3):229–35.

77. Garrigos C, Murillo O, Lora-Tamayo J, Verdaguer R, Tubau F, Cabellos C, et al. Efficacy of daptomycin-cloxacillin combination in experimental foreign-body infection due to methicillin-resistant Staphylococcus aureus. Antimicrob Agents Chemother. 2012;56(7):3806–11.

78. Garrigos C, Murillo O, Lora-Tamayo J, Verdaguer R, Tubau F, Cabellos C, et al. Fosfomycin-daptomycin and other fosfomycin combinations as alternative therapies in experimental foreign-body infection by methicillin-resistant Staphylococcus aureus. Antimicrob Agents Chemother. 2013;57(1):606–10.

79. El Haj C, Murillo O, Ribera A, Vivas M, Garcia-Somoza D, Tubau F, et al. Comparative efficacies of cloxacillin-daptomycin and the standard cloxacillin-rifampin therapies against an experimental foreign-body infection by methicillin-susceptible Staphylococcus aureus. Antimicrob Agents Chemother. 2014;58(9):5576–80.

80. El Haj C, Murillo O, Ribera A, Vivas M, Garcia-Somoza D, Tubau F, et al. Daptomycin combinations as alternative therapies in experimental foreign-body infection caused by meticillin-susceptible Staphylococcus aureus. Int J Antimicrob Agents. 2015;46(2):189–95.

81. El Haj C, Murillo O, Ribera A, Garcia-Somoza D, Tubau F, Cabellos C, et al. The anti-biofilm effect of macrolides in a rat model of S. aureus foreign-body infection: Might it be of clinical relevance? Med Microbiol Immunol. 2016;206(1):31–9. [Epub ahead of print].

82. Dhand A, Bayer AS, Pogliano J, Yang SJ, Bolaris M, Nizet V, et al. Use of antistaphylococcal beta-lactams to increase daptomycin activity in eradicating persistent bacteremia due to methicillin-resistant Staphylococcus aureus: role of enhanced daptomycin binding. Clin Infect Dis. 2011;53(2):158–63.

83. Mehta S, Singh C, Plata KB, Chanda PK, Paul A, Riosa S, et al. beta-Lactams increase the antibacterial activity of daptomycin against clinical methicillin-resistant Staphylococcus aureus strains and prevent selection of daptomycin-resistant derivatives. Antimicrob Agents Chemother. 2012;56(12):6192–200.

84. Widmer AF, Gaechter A, Ochsner PE, Zimmerli W. Antimicrobial treatment of orthopedic implant-related infections with rifampin combinations. Clin Infect Dis. 1992;14(6):1251–3.

85. Drancourt M, Stein A, Argenson JN, Zannier A, Curvale G, Raoult D. Oral rifampin plus ofloxacin for treatment of Staphylococcus-infected orthopedic implants. Antimicrob Agents Chemother. 1993;37(6):1214–8.

86. van Ingen J, Aarnoutse RE, Donald PR, Diacon AH, Dawson R, Plemper van Balen G, et al. Why do we use 600 mg of rifampicin in tuberculosis treatment? Clin Infect Dis. 2011;52(9):e194–9.

87. Kenny MT, Strates B. Metabolism and pharmacokinetics of the antibiotic rifampin. Drug Metab Rev. 1981;12(1):159–218.

88. Lora-Tamayo J, Murillo O, Ariza J. Reply to Krause et al. Clin Infect Dis. 2013;56(12):1843–4.

89. Nguyen S, Robineau O, Titecat M, Blondiaux N, Valette M, Loiez C, et al. Influence of daily dosage and frequency of administration of rifampicin-levofloxacin therapy on tolerance and effectiveness in 154 patients treated for prosthetic joint infections. Eur J Clin Microbiol Infect Dis. 2015;34(8):1675–82.

90. Hooper DC. Quinolones. In: Mandell GL, Bennett JE, Dolin R, editors. Principles & practice of infectious diseases, vol. 1. 6th ed. Philadelphia, PA: Elsevier Churchill Livingstone; 2005. p. 451–73.

91. Zhao X, Drlica K. Restricting the selection of antibiotic-resistant mutants: a general strategy derived from fluoroquinolone studies. Clin Infect Dis. 2001;33(Suppl 3):S147–56.

92. San Juan R, Garcia-Reyne A, Caba P, Chaves F, Resines C, Llanos F, et al. Safety and efficacy of moxifloxacin monother-

apy for treatment of orthopedic implant-related staphylococcal infections. Antimicrob Agents Chemother. 2010;54(12):5161–6.

93. Nijland HM, Ruslami R, Suroto AJ, Burger DM, Alisjahbana B, van Crevel R, et al. Rifampicin reduces plasma concentrations of moxifloxacin in patients with tuberculosis. Clin Infect Dis. 2007;45(8):1001–7.

94. Lora-Tamayo J, Parra-Ruiz J, Rodriguez-Pardo D, Barberan J, Ribera A, Tornero E, et al. High doses of daptomycin (10 mg/kg/d) plus rifampin for the treatment of staphylococcal prosthetic joint infection managed with implant retention: a comparative study. Diagn Micorbiol Infect Dis. 2014;80(1):66–71.

95. Morata L, Senneville E, Bernard L, Nguyen S, Buzele R, Druon J, et al. A retrospective review of the clinical experience of linezolid with or without rifampicin in prosthetic joint infections treated with debridement and implant retention. Infect Dis Ther. 2014;3(2):235–43.

96. Soriano A, Gomez J, Gomez L, Azanza JR, Perez R, Romero F, et al. Efficacy and tolerability of prolonged linezolid therapy in the treatment of orthopedic implant infections. Eur J Clin Microbiol Infect Dis. 2007;26(5):353–6.

97. Nguyen S, Pasquet A, Legout L, Beltrand E, Dubreuil L, Migaud H, et al. Efficacy and tolerance of rifampicin-linezolid compared with rifampicin-cotrimoxazole combinations in prolonged oral therapy for bone and joint infections. Clin Microbiol Infect. 2009;15(12):1163–9.

98. Drancourt M, Stein A, Argenson JN, Roiron R, Groulier P, Raoult D. Oral treatment of *Staphylococcus* spp. infected orthopaedic implants with fusidic acid or ofloxacin in combination with rifampicin. J Antimicrob Chemother. 1997;39(2):235–40.

99. Peel TN, Buising KL, Dowsey MM, Aboltins CA, Daffy JR, Stanley PA, et al. Outcome of debridement and retention in prosthetic joint infections by methicillin-resistant staphylococci, with special reference to rifampin and fusidic acid combination therapy. Antimicrob Agents Chemother. 2013;57(1):350–5.

100.Czekaj J, Dinh A, Moldovan A, Vaudaux P, Gras G, Hoffmeyer P, et al. Efficacy of a combined oral clindamycin? Rifampicin regimen for therapy of staphylococcal osteoarticular infections. Scand J Infect Dis. 2011;43(11–12):962–7.

101.Pavoni GL, Giannella M, Falcone M, Scorzolini L, Liberatore M, Carlesimo B, et al. Conservative medical therapy of prosthetic joint infections: retrospective analysis of an 8-year experience. Clin Microbiol Infect. 2004;10(9):831–7.

102. Calfee DP. Rifamycins. In: Mandell GL, Bennett JE, Dolin R, editors. Principles and practice of infectious diseases. Philadelphia, PA: Elsevier Churchill Livingstone; 2005. p. 374–88.

103. Parra-Ruiz J, Bravo-Molina A, Pena-Monje A, Hernandez-Quero J. Activity of linezolid and high-dose daptomycin, alone or in combination, in an in vitro model of Staphylococcus aureus biofilm. J Antimicrob Chemother. 2012;67(11):2682–5.

104. Steed ME, Werth BJ, Ireland CE, Rybak MJ. Evaluation of the novel combination of high-dose daptomycin plus trimethoprim-sulfamethoxazole against daptomycin-nonsusceptible methicillin-resistant Staphylococcus aureus using an in vitro pharmacokinetic/pharmacodynamic model of simulated endocardial vegetations. Antimicrob Agents Chemother. 2012;56(11):5709–14.

105. Aboltins CA, Dowsey MM, Buising KL, Peel TN, Daffy JR, Choong PF, et al. Gram-negative prosthetic joint infection treated with debridement, prosthesis retention and antibiotic regimens including a fluoroquinolone. Clin Microbiol Infect. 2011;17(6):862–7.

106. Brouqui P, Rousseau MC, Stein A, Drancourt M, Raoult D. Treatment of Pseudomonas aeruginosa-infected orthopedic prostheses with ceftazidime-ciprofloxacin antibiotic combination. Antimicrob Agents Chemother. 1995;39(11):2423–5.

107. Widmer AF, Wiestner A, Frei R, Zimmerli W. Killing of non-growing and adherent *Escherichia coli* determines drug efficacy in device-related infections. Antimicrob Agents Chemother. 1991;35(4):741–6.

108. Haagensen JA, Klausen M, Ernst RK, Miller SI, Folkesson A, Tolker-Nielsen T, et al. Differentiation and distribution of colistin- and sodium dodecyl sulfate-tolerant cells in *Pseudomonas aeruginosa* biofilms. J Bacteriol. 2007;189(1):28–37.

109. Pamp SJ, Gjermansen M, Johansen HK, Tolker-Nielsen T. Tolerance to the antimicrobial peptide colistin in *Pseudomonas aeruginosa* biofilms is linked to metabolically active cells, and depends on the pmr and mexAB-oprM genes. Mol Microbiol. 2008;68(1):223–40.

110. Corvec S, Furustrand Tafin U, Betrisey B, Borens O, Trampuz A. Activities of fosfomycin, tigecycline, colistin, and gentamicin against extended-spectrum-beta-lactamase-producing Escherichia coli in a foreign-body infection model. Antimicrob Agents Chemother. 2013;57(3):1421–7.

111. Lora-Tamayo J, Murillo O, Bergen PJ, Nation RL, Poudyal A, Luo X, et al. Activity of colistin combined with doripenem at clinically relevant concentrations against multidrug-resistant *Pseudomonas aeruginosa* in an in vitro dynamic biofilm model. J Antimicrob Chemother. 2014;69(9):2434–42.

112. Ribera A, Benavent E, Lora-Tamayo J, Tubau F, Pedrero S, Cabo X, et al. Osteoarticular infection caused by MDR *Pseudomonas aeruginosa*: the benefits of combination therapy with colistin plus beta-lactams. J Antimicrob Chemother. 2015;70(12):3357–65.

113. Olson ME, Ceri H, Morck DW, Buret AG, Read RR. Biofilm bacteria: formation and comparative susceptibility to antibiotics. Can J Vet Res. 2002;66(2):86–92.

114. Betz M, Abrassart S, Vaudaux P, Gjika E, Schindler M, Billieres J, et al. Increased risk of joint failure in hip prostheses infected with *Staphylococcus aureus* treated with debridement, antibiotics and implant retention compared to Streptococcus. Int Orthop. 2015;39(3):397–401.

115. Everts RJ, Chambers ST, Murdoch DR, Rothwell AG, McKie J. Successful antimicrobial therapy and implant retention for streptococcal infection of prosthetic joints. ANZ J Surg. 2004;74(4):210–4.

116. Meehan AM, Osmon DR, Duffy MC, Hanssen AD, Keating MR. Outcome of penicillin-susceptible streptococcal prosthetic joint infection treated with debridement and retention of the prosthesis. Clin Infect Dis. 2003;36(7):845–9.

117. Duggan JM, Georgiadis G, VanGorp C, Kleshinski J. Group B streptococcal prosthetic joint infections. J South Orthop Assoc. 2001;10(4):209–14. discussion 14.

118. Zeller V, Lavigne M, Biau D, Leclerc P, Ziza JM, Mamoudy P, et al. Outcome of group B streptococcal prosthetic hip infections compared to that of other bacterial infections. Joint Bone Spine. 2009;76(5):491–6.

119. Fiaux E, Titecat M, Robineau O, Lora-Tamayo J, El Samad Y, Etienne M, et al. Outcome of patients with streptococcal prosthetic joint infections with special reference to rifampicin combinations. BMC Infect Dis. 2016;16(1):568.

120. El Helou OC, Berbari EF, Marculescu CE, El Atrouni WI, Razonable RR, Steckelberg JM, et al. Outcome of enterococcal prosthetic joint infection: is combination systemic therapy superior to monotherapy? Clin Infect Dis. 2008;47(7):903–9.

121. Euba G, Lora-Tamayo J, Murillo O, Pedrero S, Cabo J, Verdaguer R, et al. Pilot study of ampicillin-ceftriaxone combination for treatment of orthopedic infections due to *Enterococcus faecalis*. Antimicrob Agents Chemother. 2009;53(10):4305–10.

122. Mainardi JL, Gutmann L, Acar JF, Goldstein FW. Synergistic effect of amoxicillin and cefotaxime against *Enterococcus faecalis*. Antimicrob Agents Chemother. 1995;39(9):1984–7.

123. Tornero E, Senneville E, Euba G, Petersdorf S, Rodriguez-Pardo D, Lakatos B, et al. Characteristics of prosthetic joint infections due to *Enterococcus* sp. and predictors of failure: a multinational study. Clin Microbiol Infect. 2014;20(11):1219–24.

124. Schmit JL. Efficacy of teicoplanin for enterococcal infections: 63 cases and review. Clin Infect Dis. 1992;15(2):302–6.

125. Graninger W, Wenisch C, Wiesinger E, Menschik M, Karimi J, Presterl E. Experience with outpatient intravenous teicoplanin therapy for chronic osteomyelitis. Eur J Clin Microbiol Infect Dis. 1995;14(7):643–7.

126. Falagas ME, Siempos II, Papagelopoulos PJ, Vardakas KZ. Linezolid for the treatment of adults with bone and joint infections. Int J Antimicrob Agents. 2007;29(3):233–9.

127. Yuste JR, Quesada M, Diaz-Rada P, Del Pozo JL. Daptomycin in the treatment of prosthetic joint infection by *Enterococcus faecalis*: safety and efficacy of high-dose and prolonged therapy. Int J Infect Dis. 2014;27:65–6.

128. Marculescu CE, Berbari EF, Cockerill FR 3rd, Osmon DR. Fungi, mycobacteria, zoonotic and other organisms in prosthetic joint infection. Clin Orthop Relat Res. 2006;451:64–72.

129. Phelan DM, Osmon DR, Keating MR, Hanssen AD. Delayed reimplantation arthroplasty for candidal prosthetic joint infection: a report of 4 cases and review of the literature. Clin Infect Dis. 2002;34(7):930–8.

130. Kuhn DM, George T, Chandra J, Mukherjee PK, Ghannoum MA. Antifungal susceptibility of Candida biofilms: unique efficacy of amphotericin B lipid formulations and echinocandins. Antimicrob Agents Chemother. 2002;46(6):1773–80.

131. Brooks DH, Pupparo F. Successful salvage of a primary total knee arthroplasty infected with *Candida parapsilosis*. J Arthroplast. 1998;13(6):707–12.

132. Kuiper JW, van den Bekerom MP, van der Stappen J, Nolte PA, Colen S. 2-stage revision recommended for treatment of fungal hip and knee prosthetic joint infections. Acta Orthop. 2013;84(6):517–23.

133. Berbari EF, Marculescu C, Sia I, Lahr BD, Hanssen AD, Steckelberg JM, et al. Culture-negative prosthetic joint infection. Clin Infect Dis. 2007;45(9):1113–9.

134. Malekzadeh D, Osmon DR, Lahr BD, Hanssen AD, Berbari EF. Prior use of antimicrobial therapy is a risk factor for culture-negative prosthetic joint infection. Clin Orthop Relat Res. 2010;468(8):2039–45.

135. Azzam K, McHale K, Austin M, Purtill JJ, Parvizi J. Outcome of a second two-stage reimplantation for periprosthetic knee infection. Clin Orthop Relat Res. 2009;467(7):1706–14.

136. Kubista B, Hartzler RU, Wood CM, Osmon DR, Hanssen AD, Lewallen DG. Reinfection after two-stage revision for periprosthetic infection of total knee arthroplasty. Int Orthop. 2012;36(1):65–71.

137. Mont MA, Waldman BJ, Hungerford DS. Evaluation of preoperative cultures before second-stage reimplantation of a total knee prosthesis complicated by infection. A comparison-group study. J Bone Joint Surg Am. 2000;82-A(11):1552–7.

138. Lange J, Troelsen A, Thomsen RW, Soballe K. Chronic infections in hip arthroplasties: comparing risk of reinfection following one-stage and two-stage revision: a systematic review and meta-analysis. Clin Epidemiol. 2012;4:57–73.

139. Puhto AP, Puhto TM, Niinimaki TT, Leppilahti JI, Syrjala HP. Two-stage revision for prosthetic joint infection: outcome and role of reimplantation microbiology in 107 cases. J Arthroplast. 2014;29(6):1101–4.

140. Jamsen E, Stogiannidis I, Malmivaara A, Pajamaki J, Puolakka T, Konttinen YT. Outcome of prosthesis exchange for infected knee arthroplasty: the effect of treatment approach. Acta Orthop. 2009;80(1):67–77.

141. Mahmud T, Lyons MC, Naudie DD, Macdonald SJ, McCalden RW. Assessing the gold standard: a review of 253 two-stage revisions for infected TKA. Clin Orthop Relat Res. 2012;470(10):2730–6.

142. Hoad-Reddick DA, Evans CR, Norman P, Stockley I. Is there a role for extended antibiotic therapy in a two-stage revision of the infected knee arthroplasty? J Bone Joint Surg (Br). 2005;87(2):171–4.

143. Hsieh PH, Huang KC, Lee PC, Lee MS. Two-stage revision of infected hip arthroplasty using an antibiotic-loaded spacer: retrospective comparison between short-term and prolonged antibiotic therapy. J Antimicrob Chemother. 2009;64(2):392–7.

144. Whittaker JP, Warren RE, Jones RS, Gregson PA. Is prolonged systemic antibiotic treatment essential in two-stage revision hip replacement for chronic Gram-positive infection? J Bone Joint Surg (Br). 2009;91(1):44–51.

145. Cobo J, Lora-Tamayo J, Euba G, Jover-Saenz A, Palomino J, del Toro MD, et al. Linezolid in late-chronic prosthetic joint infection caused by gram-positive bacteria. Diagn Micorbiol Infect Dis. 2013;76(1):93–8.

146. Parvizi J, Gehrke T, Musculoskeletal Infection Society. Proceedings of the International Consensus on Periprosthetic Joint Infection. 2013. http://www.msis-na.org/wp-content/themes/msis-temp/pdf/ism-periprosthetic-joint-information.pdf. Accessed 1 Jan 2017.

147. Pitto RP, Spika IA. Antibiotic-loaded bone cement spacers in two-stage management of infected total knee arthroplasty. Int Orthop. 2004;28(3):129–33.

148. Cui Q, Mihalko WM, Shields JS, Ries M, Saleh KJ. Antibiotic-impregnated cement spacers for the treatment of infection associated with total hip or knee arthroplasty. J Bone Joint Surg Am. 2007;89(4):871–82.

149. Fink B, Vogt S, Reinsch M, Buchner H. Sufficient release of antibiotic by a spacer 6 weeks after implantation in two-stage revision of infected hip prostheses. Clin Orthop Relat Res. 2011;469(11):3141–7.

150. Galvez-Lopez R, Pena-Monje A, Antelo-Lorenzo R, Guardia-Olmedo J, Moliz J, Hernandez-Quero J, et al. Elution kinetics, antimicrobial activity, and mechanical properties of 11 different antibiotic loaded acrylic bone cement. Diagn Micorbiol Infect Dis. 2014;78(1):70–4.

151. Regis D, Sandri A, Samaila E, Benini A, Bondi M, Magnan B. Release of gentamicin and vancomycin from preformed spacers in infected total hip arthroplasties: measurement of concentrations and inhibitory activity in patients' drainage fluids and serum. Sci World J. 2013;2013:752184.

152. Cabo J, Euba G, Saborido A, Gonzalez-Panisello M, Dominguez MA, Agullo JL, et al. Clinical outcome and microbiological findings using antibiotic-loaded spacers in two-stage revision of prosthetic joint infections. J Infect. 2011;63(1):23–31.

153. Kendall RW, Duncan CP, Smith JA, Ngui-Yen JH. Persistence of bacteria on antibiotic loaded acrylic depots. A reason for caution. Clin Orthop Relat Res. 1996;329:273–80.

154. Hanssen AD, Rand JA, Osmon DR. Treatment of the infected total knee arthroplasty with insertion of another prosthesis. The effect of antibiotic-impregnated bone cement. Clin Orthop Relat Res. 1994;309:44–55.

155. Westrich GH, Walcott-Sapp S, Bornstein LJ, Bostrom MP, Windsor RE, Brause BD. Modern treatment of infected total knee arthroplasty with a 2-stage reimplantation protocol. J Arthroplast. 2010;25(7):1015–21. 21 e1-2.

156. Lonner JH, Siliski JM, Della Valle C, DiCesare P, Lotke PA. Role of knee aspiration after resection of the infected total knee arthroplasty. Am J Orthop (Belle Mead NJ). 2001;30(4):305–9.

157. Atkins BL, Athanasou N, Deeks JJ, Crook DW, Simpson H, Peto TE, et al. Prospective evaluation of criteria for microbiological diagnosis of prosthetic-joint infection at revision arthroplasty. The OSIRIS Collaborative Study Group. J Clin Microbiol. 1998;36(10):2932–9.

158. Murillo O, Euba G, Calatayud L, Dominguez MA, Verdaguer R, Perez A, et al. The role of intraoperative cultures at the time of reimplantation in the management of infected total joint arthroplasty. Eur J Clin Microbiol Infect Dis. 2008;27(9):805–11.

159. Spangehl MJ, Masri BA, O'Connell JX, Duncan CP. Prospective analysis of preoperative and intraoperative investigations for the diagnosis of infection at the sites of two hundred and two revision total hip arthroplasties. J Bone Joint Surg Am. 1999;81(5):672–83.

160. Jenny JY, Lengert R, Diesinger Y, Gaudias J, Boeri C, Kempf JF. Routine one-stage exchange for chronic infection after total hip replacement. Int Orthop. 2014;38(12):2477–81.

161. Singer J, Merz A, Frommelt L, Fink B. High rate of infection control with one-stage revision of septic knee prostheses excluding MRSA and MRSE. Clin Orthop Relat Res. 2012;470(5):1461–71.

162. Tibrewal S, Malagelada F, Jeyaseelan L, Posch F, Scott G. Single-stage revision for the infected total knee replacement: results from a single centre. Bone Joint J. 2014;96-B(6):759–64.

163. Winkler H, Stoiber A, Kaudela K, Winter F, Menschik F. One stage uncemented revision of infected total hip replacement using cancellous allograft bone impregnated with antibiotics. J Bone Joint Surg (Br). 2008;90(12):1580–4.

164. Zeller V, Lhotellier L, Marmor S, Leclerc P, Krain A, Graff W, et al. One-stage exchange arthroplasty for chronic peripros-

thetic hip infection: results of a large prospective cohort study. J Bone Joint Surg Am. 2014;96(1):e1.

165. Rudelli S, Uip D, Honda E, Lima AL. One-stage revision of infected total hip arthroplasty with bone graft. J Arthroplast. 2008;23(8):1165–77.

166. Castellanos J, Flores X, Llusa M, Chiriboga C, Navarro A. The Girdlestone pseudarthrosis in the treatment of infected hip replacements. Int Orthop. 1998;22(3):178–81.

167. Corona PS, Hernandez A, Reverte-Vinaixa MM, Amat C, Flores X. Outcome after knee arthrodesis for failed septic total knee replacement using a monolateral external fixator. J Orthop Surg (Hong Kong). 2013;21(3):275–80.

168. Mabry TM, Jacofsky DJ, Haidukewych GJ, Hanssen AD. Comparison of intramedullary nailing and external fixation knee arthrodesis for the infected knee replacement. Clin Orthop Relat Res. 2007;464:11–5.

169. Haddad S, Corona PS, Reverte MM, Amat C, Flores X. Antibiotic-impregnated cement spacer as a definitive treatment for post-arthroscopy shoulder destructive osteomyelitis: case report and review of literature. Strateg Trauma Limb Reconstr. 2013;8(3):199–205.

170. Prendki V, Zeller V, Passeron D, Desplaces N, Mamoudy P, Stirnemann J, et al. Outcome of patients over 80 years of age on prolonged suppressive antibiotic therapy for at least 6 months for prosthetic joint infection. Int J Infect Dis. 2014;29:184–9.

171. Segreti J, Nelson JA, Trenholme GM. Prolonged suppressive antibiotic therapy for infected orthopedic prostheses. Clin Infect Dis. 1998;27(4):711–3.

172. Rao N, Crossett LS, Sinha RK, Le Frock JL. Long-term suppression of infection in total joint arthroplasty. Clin Orthop Relat Res. 2003;414:55–60.

173. Tsukayama DT, Wicklund B, Gustilo RB. Suppressive antibiotic therapy in chronic prosthetic joint infections. Orthopedics. 1991;14(8):841–4.

Chapter 5
Prosthetic Joint Infection: Prevention Update

Courtney Ierano, Andrew J. Stewardson, and Trisha Peel

5.1 Background

Data from the United States predict that the number of patients undergoing lower limb arthroplasty will exceed two million procedures by 2020, mirroring international predictions [1, 2]. Similar data has suggested the incidence of prosthetic joint infection is also increasing, relative to the number of procedures performed, with an estimated economic burden of

C. Ierano
National Centre for Antimicrobial Stewardship, Royal Melbourne Hospital, Parkville, Victoria, Australia

A.J. Stewardson • T. Peel (⊠)
Department of Infectious Diseases, Monash University and Alfred Health, Melbourne, Victoria, Australia
e-mail: trisha.peel@monash.edu

© Springer International Publishing AG 2018
T. Peel (ed.), *Prosthetic Joint Infections*,
https://doi.org/10.1007/978-3-319-65250-4_5

infection of $1.62 billion to US hospitals by 2020 [3]. Overall, it is estimated that approximately 55% of these infections are preventable [4]. Prevention of prosthetic joint infection is likely to lead to tangible improvement in patient outcomes in addition to cost savings for the healthcare system.

The World Health Organization (WHO) and the Centers for Disease Control and Prevention (CDC) have both recently published guidelines for prevention of surgical site infections encompassing all surgical procedures [5–7]. The WHO publication included 29 recommendations for preoperative, intra-operative and preoperative prevention of surgical site infections [6, 7]. In contrast, the Centers for Diseases Control and Prevention updated the previous publication by Mangram et al. and provided recommendations on six key questions for all procedures, in addition to recommendations for seven areas of arthroplasty [5, 8].

The scope of this chapter is therefore to review the recommendations contained in the two guidelines as they relate to the prevention of infections across the breadth of surgical practice and to examine the literature specific to the prevention of prosthetic joint infections following surgery.

5.2   Preoperative

A number of preoperative strategies have been examined for the prevention of surgical site infections. This section will touch briefly on recommendations for all surgical candidates and then focus on key areas for prevention of prosthetic joint infection including preoperative management of immuno-suppressive therapy, screening and decolonisation for *Staphylococcus aureus*, screening for asymptomatic bacteri-uria and preoperative bathing.

5.2.1   Optimisation of Comorbid Disease

As highlighted in Chap. 2, 'Epidemiology of Prosthetic Joint Infections', several co-morbid diseases have been implicated in the development of prosthetic joint infection, including obesity, malnutrition and smoking. Therefore, preoperative assessment should include attempts to optimise these risk factors. In addition, the preoperative clinical assessment should also include examination for distant infections such as urinary tract, dental or skin and soft tissue infections and to ensure that these are appropriately treated before any elective joint replacement procedure is performed [9].

5.2.2   Immunosuppressant Medications

The use of immunosuppressant medications is linked with the subsequent development of preoperative wound infections. But as noted in Chap. 2, the exact causal pathway has not been clearly delineated, and determination of whether the observed association is due to the medications or the underlying inflammatory condition, or a combination of both factors, has not been established [10].

In the WHO guidelines, there was no clear evidence to support the discontinuation of immunosuppressant medication; however, it was noted that the overall quality of evidence was poor [7]. Of interest, it was noted that analysis combining the results of two observational studies examining antitumour necrosis factor (anti-TNF) suggested that discontinuation of anti-TNF medication may be associated with a reduction in the odds of surgical site infection (OR 0.59; 95% CI 0.37–0.95) [7]. Overall, the authors of the WHO guidelines recommended that immunosuppressant therapy should not be discontinued preoperatively and cautioned about the potential risk of flare-up of the underlying inflammatory condition if the medications were ceased [7]. The CDC guidelines, when considering the question of immunosuppressant therapy specifically in prosthetic joint replacement surgery again noted the increased risk of surgical site infections with biologic agents such as anti-TNF therapy [5]. The authors noted, however, that evidence was of very low quality and that the majority of patients included in the observational studies were also receiving prednisolone, therefore potentially leading to confounding [5]. The CDC guidelines highlighted the uncertainty of current evidence regarding the potential benefits and harms of cessation of immunosuppressant therapy and were therefore unable to make recommendations on this issue. [5]. At variance with these recommendations, the International Consensus Meeting on Periprosthetic Joint Infection advocated the cessation of immunosuppressant therapy prior to joint arthroplasty, undertaken in consultation with the treating physician [11]. In the proceedings of the meeting, it was noted that there was contradictory evidence for the cessation of immunosuppressant therapy; however, the recommendation was based on expert consensus [11]. Overall, all three documents highlight the lack of definitive evidence to guide clinicians in preoperative management of immunosuppressant therapy. Clinicians should balance the potential harms of disease flare-ups with therapy cessation against the uncertain risk of surgical site infection.

In addition to systemic immunosuppressant medication, the Centers for Diseases Control and Prevention also addressed the use of intra-articular corticosteroid injections. Based on low-quality evidence drawn from review of five observational studies (two studies in knee replacement and three studies in hip replacement surgery), the authors concluded that there was no clear evidence to suggest an association between intra-articular corticosteroids and surgical site infections nor an influence of the interval of time between injections and surgery [5]. Therefore, the authors' recommendations for intra-articular corticosteroid therapy mirrored their recommendations for systemic immunosuppressant therapy [5].

5.2.3   Nasal Screening and Decolonisation
for Staphylococcus aureus

Given that S. aureus is one of the most common pathogens associated with prosthetic joint infection, the effectiveness of decolonisation in preventing infections has been well studied. S. aureus is most commonly isolated in the anterior nares;

however, it can also be isolated from other body regions including the axilla and groin. Approximately one-third of the population are colonised with *S. aureus* [12]. Colonisation with methicillin-resistant *S. aureus* is less common, but epidemiological data from the United States have suggested that the prevalence of methicillin-resistant *S. aureus* may be increasing [13]. The carriage of *S. aureus* is associated with an increased risk of surgical site infections; in a review by Kluytmans et al., the relative risk of surgical site infection was 7.1 (95% confidence interval [CI] 4.6, 11.0) for *S. aureus* carriers compared to noncarriers [12].

Studies investigating strategies to reduce *S. aureus* carriage combined approaches including detection of carriage through nasal screening and elimination of *S. aureus* using mupirocin nasal ointment with or without chlorhexidine body washes. Two early large studies demonstrated reduction in the rate of surgical site infections with intranasal mupirocin ointment; however, it did not reach statistical significance in either study [14, 15]. A subsequent systematic review by van Rijen including four studies demonstrated a 45% reduction in *S. aureus* surgical site infections with intranasal mupirocin for carriers (relative risk or risk ratio [RR] 0.55; 95% CI 0.34–0.89) [16]. This is similar to the meta-analysis conducted by the authors of the WHO guidelines, which included data from six randomised controlled trials and demonstrated a 54% reduction in the incidence of surgical site infections in patients treated with mupirocin nasal ointment (odds ratio [OR] 0.46; 95% CI 0.31, 0.69) [7]. There was an additional reduction in the incidence of other healthcare-associated infections due to *S. aureus* observed in this meta-analysis (OR 0.48; 95% CI 0.32, 0.71) emphasising that the potential benefits extend beyond preoperative wound infections [7]. The weight of evidence on the benefit of screening and decolonisation strategies exists in cardiac and orthopaedic surgery. Therefore, the WHO guideline authors recommended that patients with known colonisation with *S. aureus* undergoing cardiothoracic and orthopaedic surgery be treated preoperatively with mupirocin nasal ointment [7].

There are some important limitations to screening and decolonisation procedures. First, as noted, most carriers are colonised in the anterior nares; however, this organism can be carried on other regions of the body. In a study examining methicillin-resistant *S. aureus* carriage, use of nasal swabs alone would have failed to detect 30% of carriage in patients admitted to the intensive care unit [17]. This observation is similar to community studies for all *S. aureus* (methicillin-resistant and methicillin-susceptible) carriage: in a study by Young et al., 27.5% of *S. aureus* carriage was detected on swabs from sites other than the nose [18]. In addition, approximately 60% of the population intermittently carry *S. aureus*; therefore, it may not be present at the time of screening or may be missed if only the anterior nares are sampled [12]. The efficacy of screening and decolonisation may not be absolute. In a study by Baratz et al., 22% of patients with methicillin-resistant *S. aureus* detected on preoperative screening of the anterior nares had the same organism isolated on repeat sampling on the day of surgery despite undergoing decolonisation with mupirocin and chlorhexidine body washes [19]. Repeat screening for methicillin-resistant *S. aureus* was only performed on those patients who were positive on the initial screening. There are limitations to this study. First, patients did not undergo screening following decolonisation to document clearance; therefore, it is unclear whether the cases detected on repeat screening represent a failure of decolonisation or reacquisition of this organism. Second, only the anterior nares were swabbed [19]. In a study by Harbarth et al. examining universal screening for methicillin-resistant *S. aureus* in surgical departments at the University of Geneva hospitals, 57% of patients who developed a staphylococcal infection during the hospital admission had negative admission screening swabs (which consisted of anterior nares and perineal swabs) [20]. The intermittent nature of carriage or carriage of *S. aureus* at a site other than the nares or perineum may account for the observations by Harbarth et al. and Baratz et al. Alternatively, as postulated by Harbarth et al., alternate methods of transmission, including nosocomial transmission, may account for the pre-operative acquisition of infection with *S. aureus* [20]. Therefore, prevention of *S. aureus* surgical site infection cannot rely on screening and decolonisation strategies alone but must be implemented in parallel with other infection prevention strategies, such as hand hygiene.

The other concern with *S. aureus* decolonisation is the potential for emergence of resistance to mupirocin. In the systematic review by van Rijen et al., mupirocin resistance was documented in <0.6% of the study populations, and there was no clear association between mupirocin use and the emergence resistance to this agent [16]. The overall rate of mupirocin resistance was higher among patients in a large cluster randomised controlled trial (REDUCE-MRSA trial) examining decolonisation strategies for methicillin-resistant *S. aureus* in intensive care units; the overall rate of mupirocin resistance was higher in these patients, which may reflect the differences in study populations [21]. Overall 7.5% of methicillin-resistant *S. aureus* isolates exhibited high-level resistance to mupirocin, and consistent with van Rijen et al., this did not change significantly with the use of mupirocin compared to the control arm [21]. Mupirocin resistance appears uncommon outside of the intensive care unit, and there is no clear association between mupirocin use and emergence of resistance. It remains a concern, however, and warrants ongoing monitoring, particularly in settings with universal mupirocin application [22].

5.2.4   Screening and Treatment of Asymptomatic Bacteriuria

Pre- and postoperative infections at extra-articular sites have been implicated in the development of prosthetic joint infection in epidemiological studies [23, 24]. In an early observational study by Surin et al., patients who were diagnosed with an extra-articular infection, the majority of whom had urinary tract infections, were three times more likely to develop prosthetic joint infection (calculated RR 2.7; 95% CI 1.3–5.7) [25]. It was hypothesised that remote infections could cause haematogenous seeding of the prosthesis leading to a prosthetic joint infection. Surin et al. noted, however, that there was no correlation between causative agents of the extra-articular infection and the microorganism ultimately isolated from the infected prosthesis [25]. In a subsequent large prospective observational study by Sousa et al., all patients underwent screening for asymptomatic bacteriuria prior to joint replacement surgery [26]. Treatment of asymptomatic bacteriuria cases was undertaken at the discretion of the treating clinician. Overall, 12.1% of patients had bacteria detected on preoperative screening, and the risk of subsequent prosthetic joint infection was higher in these patients (OR 3.23; 95% CI 1.67–6.27) [26]. In keeping with prior observations, the organisms isolated at preoperative urine screening were distinct from those isolated from infected prosthetic joints [26]. The authors also noted that patients with asymptomatic bacteriuria were more likely to be older, female and obese and have a higher American Society of Anesthesiologists score, raising the possibility that the presence of bacteriuria may represent a surrogate marker or confounder rather than true causality [26]. In addition, the treatment of asymptomatic bacteriuria did not reduce the incidence of prosthetic joint infection [26]. A randomised trial by Cordero-Ampuero et al. examines whether treatment of asymptomatic bacteriuria prevented subsequent prosthetic joint infections. In this study, patients with asymptomatic bacteriuria detected on preoperative screening were randomly assigned to either receive antibiotic therapy directed against the isolated bacteria or no treatment [27]. There was no difference in the risk of prosthetic joint infection between the groups (calculated RR 1.2; 95% CI 0.4–3.6) [27]. This study may not be considered definitive, however, given the lack of blinding, potential selection bias and low power.

There are few studies examining the cost-effectiveness of preoperative urinalysis. In a study examining 'non-prosthetic' knee surgery, Lawrence et al. noted that the costs of screening exceeded the cost of treatment of any infection and therefore concluded that preoperative urinalysis was unlikely to be cost-effective. The authors extrapolated their findings to other surgical types, including joint replacement surgery, drawing the same conclusions [28]. In addition to the uncertain cost-benefit of urinalysis and treatment of asymptomatic bacteriuria, of greater concern is the ecological impact of this practice, in particular, the emergence of antimicrobial resistance. The treatment of asymptomatic bacteriuria is consistently discouraged by national and international guidelines. Given these concerns and the lack of clear causal pathways, the preoperative screening for asymptomatic bacteriuria is not well supported by the literature. In the Proceedings of the International Consensus Meeting, it was recommended that routine urine urinalysis should not be performed in patients without overt symptoms of a urinary tract infection [11].

5.2.5   Preoperative Bathing

The role of preoperative bathing or showering has been examined in several settings without clear evidence to support its efficacy. A large Cochrane review conducted by Webster et al. in 2015 included 10,000 patients from seven randomised controlled trials [29]. The review included one trial comparing preoperative bathing with 4% chlorhexidine gluconate to placebo, one trial comparing preoperative bathing with 4% chlorhexidine gluconate to nonmedicated soap and three trials comparing preoperative bathing with 4% chlorhexidine gluconate to either nonmedicated soap or placebo [29]. There was no evidence to support preoperative bathing with 4% chlorhexidine gluconate compared with either placebo or nonmedicated soap for the prevention of surgical site infections (Figs. 5.1 and 5.2) [29].

The authors noted a number of methodological issues with some of the trials including limited participant follow-up and limited data on costs or cost-effectiveness [29].

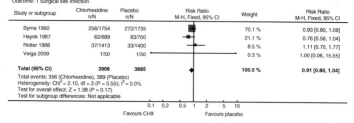

FIGURE 5.1 Comparison of 4% chlorhexidine gluconate to placebo (From Webster and Osborne [29], with permission)

Review: Preoperative bathing or showering with skin antiseptics to prevent surgical site infection
Comparison: 2 Chlorhexidine 4% versus bar soap
Outcome: 1 Surgical site infection

Study or subgroup	Chlorhexidine 4% n/N	Bar soap n/N	Risk Ratio M-H, Random, 95% CI	Weight	Risk Ratio M-H, Random, 95% CI
Earnshaw 1989	8/31	4/35		19.0 %	2.26 [0.75, 6.77]
Hayek 1987	62/689	80/626		48.6 %	0.70 [0.51, 0.96]
Randall 1983	12/32	10/30		32.4 %	1.13 [0.57, 2.21]
Total (95% CI)	**752**	**691**		**100.0 %**	**1.02 [0.57, 1.84]**

Total events: 82 (Chlorhexidine 4%), 94 (Bar soap)
Heterogeneity: Tau² = 0.16, Chi² = 5.02, df = 2 (P = 0.08); I² = 60%
Test for overall effect: Z = 0.07 (P = 0.94)
Test for subgroup differences: Not applicable

0.01   0.1   1   10   100
Favours CHX   Favours bar soap

FIGURE 5.2 Comparison of 4% chlorhexidine to nonmedicated soap (From Webster and Osborne [29], with permission

The meta-analysis undertaken as part of the recent WHO guidelines included two observational studies in addition to seven randomised controlled trials examining chlorhexidine gluconate to nonmedicated soap. As with the findings in the Cochrane review, preoperative bathing with chlorhexidine gluconate did not significantly reduce the odds of surgical site infections (combined OR 0.92; 95% CI 0.80–1.04) [7]. Similar conclusion was drawn in the CDC guidelines [5]. Both guidelines noted that bathing or showering preoperatively was an accepted practice; however, there was no conclusive evidence to support the use of chlorhexidine over nonmedicated soap [5, 7].

There are also significant concerns with patient compliance with preoperative chlorhexidine bathing [30]. In addition, application and subsequent rinsing of the chlorhexidine may result in lower delivery of the antiseptic and may impact the residual activity of chlorhexidine [31]. Given these concerns, recent interest has focused on the role of chlorhexidine-impregnated wipes or cloths, including in patient undergoing joint replacement surgery [30, 32, 33]. The WHO guidelines also included meta-analysis data on the use of these wipes based on three low-quality observational studies. The risk of surgical site infections was reduced with chlorhexidine-impregnated cloths (OR 0.27; 95% CI 0.09–0.79). These results are similar to those reported in a systematic review by Karki et al. which examined the impact of chlorhexidine-impregnated wipes for prevention of health-care-associated infections [31]. This systematic review included one randomised controlled trial and four observational studies in patients undergoing surgery. The use of chlorhexidine-impregnated wipes was associated with a 71% reduction in the risk of surgical site infection on pooled analysis (RR 0.29; 95% CI 0.17–0.49) [31]. As with the WHO analysis, the studies including this systematic review were of low quality. Given the limitations of current evidence, the WHO concluded there was insufficient evidence to provide a recommendation on the use of chlorhexidine-impregnated cloths [7]. Similarly the use of chlorhexidine-impregnated cloths was considered an unresolved issue in the CDC guidelines [5].

5.2.6   Hair Removal

The removal of hair from the planned operative site was traditionally performed as it was thought to increase the efficacy of skin antisepsis and aid with dressing adherence and integrity. However, recent systematic reviews have indicated that preoperative hair removal may be associated with an increased risk of surgical site infections [8]. In particular, shaving is thought to increase the risk of surgical site infections due to microscopic cuts that compromise skin integrity [8]. A recent Cochrane review undertaken by Tanner et al., included four randomised controlled trials and ten quasi-randomised controlled trials comparing shaving with clippers ($n = 1$), shaving with depilatory creams ($n = 6$) and shaving with no hair removal ($n = 4$) and one trial compared shaving with clippers or no hair removal and one trial compared shaving with depilatory cream or no hair removal. The final trial examined hair removal with clippers or shaving at different times in the perioperative period [34]. They found no increased risk of surgical site infections with shaving compared to no hair removal (Fig. 5.3).

Only one trial was included in the analysis examining clipping to no hair removal (Fig. 5.4). There was no difference in the risk of surgical site infections; however, the number included was small ($n = 130$) and the confidence interval was broad [34].

Similarly, there was no difference when depilatory cream was compared to no hair removal (RR 1.02; 95% CI 0.45–2.31) [34]. However, when the authors compared shaving to clipping, the risk of surgical site infections was higher with shaving compared to clipping (RR 2.03; 95% CI 1.14–3.61) (Fig. 5.5) [34]. This was predominantly influenced by a single trial by Alexander et al., a randomised trial including patients

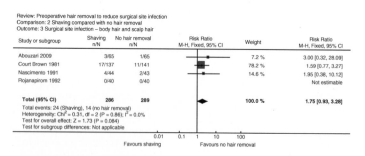

FIGURE 5.3 Comparison of shaving to no hair removal (From Tanner et al. [34], with permission)

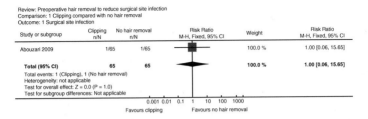

FIGURE 5.4 Comparison of clipping to no hair removal (From Tanner et al. [34], with permission)

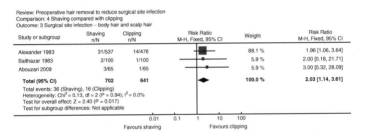

FIGURE 5.5 Comparison of shaving to clipping (From Tanner et al. [34], with permission)

undergoing a range of surgical procedures (it is unclear whether elective joint replacement surgery was included in the cohort) with four arms comparing clipping in the evening before or the morning of surgery or shaving in the evening before or morning of surgery [35]. Of note, the Cochrane review included cases of stitch abscess in the total number of infections; these stitch abscesses were specifically excluded by Alexander et al. as they are not considered a surgical site infection when the CDC definition was applied [8, 35]. In the original study, there were 25 infections among 537 patients (4.6%) in the shaving group compared to 13 infections among 516 patients (2.5%) in the clipping group (RR 1.89; 95% CI 0.98–3.66; $P = 0.06$) [35].

In the subsequent meta-analysis in the WHO guidelines, the association between clipping and shaving was supported.

Overall clipping was associated with a 49% reduction in surgical site infections compared to shaving (OR 0.51; 95% CI 0.34–0.78) [7]. Therefore, hair should ideally not be removed, or if removal is necessary, then clipping is advised [7].

5.3   Operative

At the time of surgery, several strategies have been associated with a lower risk of surgical site infection across a range of surgical specialities. These strategies include attention to physiological homeostasis, reduction in bacterial skin and wound contamination using antisepsis and antimicrobial prophylaxis, wound closure techniques and attention to the operating room environment and theatre discipline.

5.3.1   Physiological Homeostasis

The recently published WHO and CDC guidelines included some overlapping recommendations for glycaemic control, maintenance of normal body temperature (normothermia) intraoperatively and intraoperative oxygenation targets.

With respect to glycaemic control, the WHO guidelines noted from a review of 15 randomised controlled trials that intensive perioperative glycaemic control was associated with a 57% reduction in the odds of surgical site infections (OR 0.43; 95% CI 0.29–0.64) in patients with and without diabetes mellitus; however, the optimal threshold glucose concentrations were not established [6]. While cautioning about the potential adverse impact of hypoglycaemia, the authors made a conditional recommendation for intensive perioperative glycaemic control supported by low quality of evidence [6]. In contrast, the CDC guidelines recommended perioperative glycaemic control with targets of less than 200 mg/dL for both diabetic and nondiabetic patients [5]. This was graded as a strong recommendation based on high- to moderate-quality evidence derived from two randomised trials in cardiac surgery [5]. While both guidelines emphasised the importance of glycaemic control for both diabetic and nondiabetic patients, the optimal threshold for glucose concentrations appears to be an unresolved issue with divergent literature [5, 6].

With respect to oxygenation, both guidelines included strong recommendation based on moderate-quality evidence about the administration of increased fraction of inspired oxygen (FiO_2) [5, 6]. The administration of high FiO_2 (80%) was associated with a 27% reduction in the odds of surgical site infections compared to standard FiO_2 (OR 0.72; 95% CI 0.55–0.94). Similarly, there was agreement with respect to maintenance of normal body temperature (normothermia) considered a strong recommendation based on analysis of two randomised controlled trials [5, 6].

5.3.2   Surgical Hand Preparation

Surgical hand antisepsis to remove transient flora and reduce resident skin flora is considered standard practice in preparation for surgery. The two recommended methods are surgical hand scrubbing with antimicrobial soap and water and surgical handrubbing with a waterless alcohol-based handrub [36]. There is limited evidence regarding which is the optimal agent for surgical hand preparation.

In a meta-analysis by Tanner et al., two aspects of surgical hand preparation were examined: firstly, the impact of surgical hand preparation on surgical site infections and the impact of different agents on the number of bacteria present on the surgeon's hands following cleansing [36]. Four randomised trials examining the impact of surgical hand antisepsis on surgical site infections were identified and included in the meta-analysis. The included studies were noted be of low or moderate quality and included a variety of active components and approaches, limiting comparison. Overall, no trial demonstrated superiority of one agent or approach for the prevention of surgical site infections [36].

Ten studies examine the impact of surgical hand antisepsis on the number of bacteria present on the skin, measured as the number of colony-forming units (CFUs). Again the authors noted low to moderate quality of evidence with noted methodological issues identified [36]. Chlorhexidine gluconate was associated with a reduced number of CFUs compared with povidone-iodine, and the effect was sustained out to 2 h following scrubbing (Fig. 5.6). However, these studies did not examine the clinical impact of this observation, in particular whether this observed reduction in hand contamination was associated with fewer surgical site infections [36]. In addition, among the four studies comparing surgical handrubbing to surgical handwashing, there was a suggestion that alcohol-based handrubs were more effective at reducing CFUs. But due to study quality, the authors were reticent to draw definitive conclusions [36].

In the meta-analysis performed in the WHO guidelines, similar conclusions were drawn: namely, while surgical hand preparation was an accepted aspect of overall patient care, there was no evidence to support one method or agent over a comparator [7].

Review: Surgical hand antisepsis to reduce surgical site infection
Comparison: 2 chlorhexidine versus iodine
Outcome: 1 CFUs

Study or subgroup	Chlorhexidine N	Mean (SD)	Iodine N	Mean (SD)	Mean Difference IV, Fixed, 95% CI	Mean Difference IV, Fixed, 95% CI
1. CFUs immediately after antisepsis						
Furukawa 2005	11	0.1 (0.4)	11	2.5 (1.4)		−2.40 [−3.26, −1.54]
Herruzo 2000	50	18 (6)	49	66 (7)		−48.00 [−50.57, −45.43]
Pereira 1990	34	3.99 (0.7)	34	4.33 (0.56)		−0.34 [−0.64, −0.04]
Pereira 1990	34	4.11 (0.23)	34	4.28 (0.23)		−0.17 [−0.28, −0.06]
2. CFUs 2 h after initial antisepsis						
Pereira 1990	34	3.6 (0.64)	34	4.35 (0.65)		−0.75 [−1.06, −0.44]
Pereira 1990	34	3.83 (0.56)	34	4.24 (0.74)		−0.41 [−0.72, −0.10]
3. CFUs 2 h after subsequent antisepsis						
Pereira 1990	34	3.44 (0.81)	34	4.54 (0.48)		−1.10 [−1.42, −0.78]
Pereira 1990	34	4.02 (0.63)	34	4.67 (0.54)		−0.65 [−0.93, −0.37]
4. CFUs after surgical procedure						
Herruzo 2000	50	37 (11)	49	169 (31)		−132.00 [−141.20, −122.80]

−1   −0.5   0   0.5   1
Favours Chlorhex   Favours Iodine

FIGURE 5.6 Comparison of number of CFUs present over time following surgical hand antisepsis with chlorhexidine gluconate or povidone iodine scrubs (From Tanner et al. [36], with permission)

5.3.3   *Surgical Skin Preparation*

In addition to the potential contamination of the surgical incision with bacteria from the hands of the healthcare worker, the patient's own skin flora is thought to be a major source of bacterial contamination of the surgical site [37, 38]. This bacterial contamination may lead to surgical site infection, and procedures in which prosthetic material are implanted, such as joint replacement surgery, are particularly prone to infection. In a rabbit model study by Southwood et al., the infectious dose of *S. aureus* required to establish an infection in 50% (ID_{50}) of animals was 200-fold higher in the absence of prosthetic material. Indeed contamination of the prosthesis with only 50 *S. aureus* bacteria at the time of implantation induced an infection in 50% of the animals tested [39].

Preoperative skin antisepsis is performed in the operating room and aims to reduce the microbial load on the patient's skin prior to the surgical incision [7]. The three agents commonly used for skin antisepsis are chlorhexidine gluconate, iodophors or alcohol [40]. Alcohol acts rapidly to denature the cell wall protein of a range of microorganisms, but it has no residual activity [41, 42]. Chlorhexidine gluconate is bactericidal and acts through disruption of the outer cell membranes and cytoplasmic membranes of microorganisms [42]. It has a slower onset of action, but it has prolonged residual activity [8, 43]. Iodine is frequently formulated in a polyvinylpyrrolidone-iodine (povidone-iodine) complex which improves the stability of iodine and allows for slower release of free iodine [8, 41, 42]. Iodine disrupts intracellular proteins in microorganisms [42]. Iodophors are inactivated by organic material, including blood and serum which may impact their efficacy [8, 40]. They have minimal residual activity, but they exhibit persistence of bacteriostatic activity when on the skin [8]. Alcohol is frequently combined with chlorhexidine gluconate or iodophors to augment the activity of these agents [40]. Guidelines frequently recommend against the sequential application of iodophors after chlorhexidine as it is theorised that iodophors may inactivate chlorhexidine [38, 44]. However, this has not been supported by in vitro studies: indeed, in a study by Anderson et al., the activity of chlorhexidine gluconate and povidone-iodine was augmented when used in combination [43]. There are limited clinical studies examining the combination of chlorhexidine and povidone-iodine; two cohort studies in patients undergoing neurosurgical procedures have examined these combinations, but there are no randomised controlled trials to date [45, 46].

The optimal agent for skin antisepsis has been the focus of significant research interest. Despite this, a meta-analysis by Dumville et al. in 2015 was unable to provide definitive evidence of superiority of one agent, owing in part to the paucity of high-quality, adequately powered trials [41]. In the meta-analysis performed in the WHO guidelines, alcohol-based antiseptic combinations were compared with aqueous-based preparations. Analysis of twelve randomised controlled trials demonstrated the use of alcohol-based preparations was associated with a 40% reduction in the risk of surgical site infections (OR 0.60; 95% CI 0.45–0.78) [7]. There was low- to moderate-quality evidence suggesting chlorhexidine-alcohol combinations were superior to iodophor-alcohol-based combinations (OR 0.58; 95% CI 0.42–0.80) [7]. Based on these analyses, the WHO guidelines recommended the use of alcohol-based chlorhexidine gluconate antiseptic solutions for skin preparation [7].

In contrast, the CDC guidelines did not demonstrate benefit of chlorhexidine-alcohol combinations over iodophor-alcohol combinations based on the analysis of six randomised controlled trials with high grade of evidence base (OR 0.64; 95% CI 0.24–1.71) [5]. Therefore, while concurring with the need for an alcohol-based antiseptic, the CDC guidelines did not include a specific recommendation for use of chlorhexidine or iodophor [5].

Overall there is an agreement that alcohol-based preparations are optimal, but there remains conflicting data and recommendations about whether chlorhexidine gluconate or an iodophor is the superior agent to use in combination with alcohol.

Given the known association between shoulder surgery and *Cutibacterium acnes* (formerly known as *Propionibacterium acnes*) surgical site infections, a number of research groups have examined the efficacy of surgical antiseptic preparations against this organism. In a study by Saltzman et al., 150 patients were randomised to surgical antiseptic preparation with either chlorhexidine gluconate and alcohol, iodophor and alcohol or iodine scrub and paint. The surgical incision site was swabbed following skin preparation, and the rate of positive cultures for different microorganisms was compared. Coagulase-negative *Staphylococcus* species and *C. acnes* were the most common isolates [47]. When comparing the alcohol-based solutions, an organism was isolated in 19% of cases when iodophor-alcohol were used compared with 7% of cases with chlorhexidine-alcohol ($P = 0.01$): there was no difference observed with respect to the isolation of *C. acnes*; however, the number of isolates was small ($n = 28$) [47]. There were no surgical site infections observed in this study; therefore, the clinical impact of the observed difference could not be assessed [47]. A similar study by Savage et al. in lumbar surgery did not find significant difference in rates of positive cultures after skin preparation or wound closure with alcohol-based chlorhexidine preparations compared with alcohol-based iodine preparations [48]. *C. acnes* has a predilection for deeper dermal structures such as sebaceous glands; therefore, Lee et al. postulated that the failure of skin preparation to eliminate *C. acnes* in the dermis may act as the potential source of this bacteria in shoulder joint surgical site infections [49]. Dermal punch biopsies were obtained in ten healthy male volunteers following skin antisepsis with an alcohol-based chlorhexidine solution and cultured for *C. acnes*. *C. acnes* was isolated in 70% of dermal specimens, despite skin antisepsis [49]. In a follow-up from these observations, Sabetta et al. examined whether the preoperative application of benzoyl peroxide, a commonly used topical preparation for acne treatment, would lead to a reduction in culture positivity for *C. acnes* [50]. Using the untreated (with benzoyl peroxide), nonsurgical arm as control, Sabetta et al. observed a significant reduction in the number of positive cultures isolating *C. acnes* [50]. Once again, the clinical implications of these observational studies have not been established and further investigation is required.

5.3.4 Adhesive Drapes

Plastic, adhesive, incise drapes are commonly used in surgery based on a theoretical risk of contamination of the wound by skin flora and the thought that the adhesive drapes act as a 'microbial barrier' [51]. However, a number of studies have raised concerns as to whether the presence of adhesive drapes may promote bacterial growth and, therefore, conversely increase the risk of surgical site infection [52, 53]. A randomised controlled trial by Falk-Brynhildsen et al. examined bacterial recolonisation of the skin with adhesive drapes in 140 patients undergoing cardiac surgery [52]. Significant differences were observed in the proportion of skin swabs recolonised with *C. acnes* when adhesive drapes were used compared to no drapes after 120 min (63.1% versus 44.4%, respectively; $P = 0.034$), and also an increased proportion of subcutaneous tissue specimens isolated coagulase-negative staphylococci at the end of surgery in patients with adhesive drapes (14.7% versus 4.5%, respectively; $P = 0.044$) [52].

This question was recently addressed in a Cochrane review by Webster et al. [51]. The initial analysis compared the incidence of surgical site infections with and without adhesive drapes in a range of surgical procedures. Five randomised controlled trials with 3082 participants were included, and the analysis demonstrated an increased risk of infection with adhesive drapes (RR 1.23; 95% CI 1.02–1.48) with high-quality evidence [51]. The second analysis compared iodine-impregnated adhesive drapes compared to no adhesive drapes and included two randomised controlled trials with 1133 participants. The pooled analysis did not demonstrate any increased risk of infection with iodine-impregnated drapes (RR 1.03; 95% CI 0.66–1.60) with moderate-quality evidence [51].

In contrast, the meta-analysis conducted by Berríos-Torres et al. in the CDC guidelines did not demonstrate an increased risk of infection with the use of drapes compared with no drapes (n = 1,742, RR 1.05; 95% CI 0.66–1.60) [5]. This meta-analysis included four randomised controlled trials (which were also included in the Cochrane review); however, the meta-analysis did not include the study by Cordtz et al., which was included in the review by Webster et al. [5, 51]. Cordtz et al. conducted a factorial randomised controlled trial in 1340 patients undergoing caesarean section comparing incision drape or no drape with or without skin disinfection with 2.5% iodine in 70% alcohol [54]. The frequency of infections was higher in patients with adhesive drapes (15.0% versus 10.9%; RR 1.37; 95% CI 1.03–1.82) [51, 54]. When examining iodine-impregnated drapes, Berríos-Torres et al. identified the same two randomised controlled trials as Webster et al. with similar results [5, 51]. The CDC recommended that adhesive drapes were not necessary to prevent surgical site infections as a weak recommendation [5]. Webster et al. agreed with the conclusion that there was no evidence to support the use of drapes adding that nonimpregnated may increase the risk of infection [51].

5.3.5   Surgical Antimicrobial Prophylaxis

Optimal surgical antimicrobial prophylaxis prescribed requires adoption of seven key principles (Table 5.1). In regard to joint replacement surgery, the specific literature regarding these elements is quite broad in terms of quality. The current literature predominantly references hip and knee joint replacement surgery as opposed to elbow, ankle and shoulder arthroplasty. However, the evidence pertaining to the surgical antimicrobial principles for lower limb joint replacement surgery can be broadly applied to arthroplasty in general.

Joint replacement surgery is classified as a class I/clean procedure by the CDC surgical wound classification system, but given that the procedure involves the implantation of foreign material, surgical antimicrobial prophylaxis is recommended [8, 55].

TABLE 5.1 Principles of surgical antimicrobial prophylaxis prescribing (Data from Bratzler et al. [55])

Right indication	Prescription of surgical antimicrobial prophylaxis for procedures where there is evidence to support its use
Right antimicrobial	The antimicrobial selected targets the most common organisms causing infections, avoiding unnecessary broad-spectrum antimicrobials where possible
Right route	The antimicrobial is administered by the most efficacious route to maximise effect
Right dose	The dose given is adequate to ensure optimal levels of activity against the most commonly isolated microorganisms associated with surgical site infections
Right timing	The antimicrobial is administered at the optimal time to ensure maximal levels of the drug are present in the incision site tissues at the time of the procedure
Right intraoperative dosing	In antimicrobials with a short half-life (such as cefazolin), repeat doses are administered as required, to ensure optimal levels of the antimicrobial are present in the tissues throughout the procedure
Right duration	The length of time the antimicrobials are administered in the perioperative and postoperative period is supported by evidence balancing the risk of surgical site infections with unintended harms from antimicrobial exposure, including risk of *Clostridium difficile*

Indication   Multiple systematic reviews and meta-analyses have been conducted over the last decade regarding the use of prophylactic antimicrobials for hip and knee joint replacement procedures and support the principle of prophylactic antimicrobial use to reduce surgical site infections [56–58].

An early meta-analysis, AlBuhairan et al. pooled the data from seven randomised controlled trials and demonstrated that the use of antimicrobial prophylaxis was associated with an 81% risk of wound infection compared with no antibiotics among patients undergoing arthroplasty (RR 0.19; 95% CI 0.12–0.31) [58]. This included studies in which the prophylaxis was administered in the form of antibiotic-loaded cement with or without intravenous antimicrobials. In addition, the authors conducted multiple pooled analyses and did not identify any significant difference when comparing the following: cephalosporins with teicoplanin (RR 1.22; 95% CI 0.64–2.34), cephalosporins with penicillin derivatives (RR 1.17; 95% CI 0.31–4.41) and second-generation with first-generation cephalosporins (RR 1.08; 95% CI 0.63–1.84) [58]. It is important to note that the studies included in these pooled analyses ranged from 1979 to 1999 [58]. The authors also highlighted a number of methodological issues impacting on the quality and interpretation of the included trials [58].

In a subsequent meta-analysis in primary hip and knee joint replacement by Voigt et al., the use of systemic intravenous surgical antimicrobial prophylaxis was associated with a 77% reduction in the risk of infection after 6–12 months of follow-up compared to placebo (RR 0.23; 95% CI 0.12–0.43) [56]. Similar findings were demonstrated when assessing infections in the longer term (up to 6.5 years). However, this pooled analysis was for primary hip joint replacements, and all included studies were of moderate grade quality [56].

Antimicrobial   The decision regarding the best antimicrobial agent for surgical prophylaxis needs to take into account the likely pathogens encountered while being cognisant of potential toxicities and costs of the antimicrobial agent [55]. As noted in Chap. 2, 'Epidemiology of Prosthetic Joint Infections' (Table 2.1), coagulase-negative *Staphylococcus* and *S. aureus* are the predominant organisms isolated in prosthetic joint infections, with aerobic Gram-negative bacilli being the third most common isolates. Therefore, the optimal agent selected should be active against these organisms. For the majority of procedures, a first-generation cephalosporin, such as cefazolin, is the preferred drug of choice for surgical antimicrobial prophylaxis [55]. However, several studies have evaluated whether glycopeptide antibiotics, such as vancomycin or teicoplanin, are indicated in centres with a high prevalence of methicillin-resistant *Staphylococcus* [59, 60].

Vancomycin has been studied as a prophylactic antibiotic in randomised controlled trials in cardiothoracic surgery including a study by Finkelstein et al., in which vancomycin was compared to cefazolin in patients undergoing sternotomy. Overall there was a 73% reduction in methicillin-resistant *S. aureus* and 82% reduction in *Enterococcus*. There was, however, a significant increase in methicillin-susceptible *S. aureus* in patients receiving vancomycin [61]. Data from the Victorian Healthcare Associated Surveillance System, in Australia, by Bull et al. have identified a similar trend [62]. In this large retrospective observational study, including 10,973 hip and 7369 knee joint replacement surgeries, there was a significant increase in methicillin-susceptible *S. aureus* in patients receiving vancomycin alone as surgical antimicrobial prophylaxis compared with beta-lactam antibiotics [62].

A systematic review and meta-analysis were performed by Saleh and colleagues comparing glycopeptide and beta-lactam surgical antibiotic prophylaxis in cardiovascular and orthopaedic surgery [63]. Overall fourteen randomised controlled trials were included in the meta-analysis; including six studies examining patients undergoing orthopaedic procedures. No included trial examined combination prophylaxis with a beta-lactam plus a glycopeptide antimicrobial. There was no difference in the overall incidence of surgical site infections between glycopeptide and beta-lactam surgical antimicrobial prophylaxis (RR 0.87; 95% CI 0.63–1.18; $P = 0.37$). There was, however, a reduction in the incidence of methicillin-resistant staphylococcal infections (RR 0.52; 95% CI 0.29–0.93) and enterococcal infections (RR 0.36; 95% CI 0.16–0.80) with glycopeptide surgical antimicrobial prophylaxis [63]. Therefore, current data does not demonstrate an overall efficacy with vancomycin when used alone. Indeed, data suggest that use of vancomycin in isolation may conversely lead to an increase in methicillin-susceptible *S. aureus* surgical site infections.

Based on these observations, the potential benefit of combination prophylaxis to cover both sensitive and resistant staphylococci is currently being examined. A Cochrane review examined surgical antimicrobial prophylaxis for prevention of methicillin-resistant *S. aureus* surgical site infections following other surgical procedures. The review included twelve randomised controlled trials, including two studies examining combination surgical antimicrobial prophylaxis. The authors could not draw definitive conclusions about the role of combination surgical antimicrobial prophylaxis, due to the high risk of bias, very low quality of evidence, significant heterogeneity and lack of patient and economic outcome data. The authors concluded that there was a need for well-designed randomised controlled trial in this arena [64].

In the absence of such a trial, there is evidence from observational studies demonstrating a reduction in the incidence of infections after introduction of combination prophylaxis in total joint replacement surgery [65–68]. A retrospective review of 1828 patients by Sewick et al. compared the efficacy of a combination antibiotic prophylaxis regimen (cefazolin and vancomycin) to cefazolin alone [69]. Infection rates were comparable, 1.1% and 1.4%, respectively; methicillin-resistant *S. aureus* infections were reduced when comparing the combination prophylaxis to the cefazolin regimens, 0.008% and 0.8%, respectively ($P = 0.022$) [69]. However, the number needed to treat with additional vancomycin prophylaxis to prevent one methicillin-resistant *S. aureus* infection was high (138, 95% CI: 101.5–2828.2) [69].

Similarly, Liu et al. examined the role of combination prophylaxis with vancomycin and cefazolin in 414 patients undergoing revision hip or knee replacement surgery. The introduction of combination prophylaxis reduced the rate of infection from 7.89% to 3.13% (Fisher's exact test $P = 0.046$)

[67]. The proportion of methicillin-resistant *Staphylococcus* decreased from 53% to 29% following introduction [67].

A third group examined the incidence of prosthetic joint infection after the introduction of combination prophylaxis with teicoplanin and cefuroxime in a retrospective cohort of 1896 patients undergoing total hip or knee arthroplasty. Tornero et al. reported a 64% reduction in the overall risk of prosthetic joint infection following the adoption combination prophylaxis (hazard ratio 0.355; 95% CI 0.170–0.740). There was a significant reduction in infections due to Gram-positive bacteria following the introduction of combination prophylaxis (2.9% versus 0.9%; $P = 0.002$). In particular, there was a reduction in both methicillin-susceptible and methicillin-resistant *S. aureus* infection in the combination prophylaxis cohort (1.6% to 0%; $P < 0.0001$) [68].

The reduction in the incidence of surgical site infections must be balanced against the potential unintended consequences of combination surgical antimicrobial prophylaxis. These concerns include serious adverse outcomes such as acute kidney injury, reported by Courtney et al. following the introduction of combination surgical antimicrobial prophylaxis (13% versus 8% for cefazolin prophylaxis; $P = 0.002$) [70]. Another major concern with vancomycin prophylaxis is the emergence of vancomycin-resistant *Enterococcus* (VRE) and other antibiotic-resistant microorganisms [71]. Exposure to vancomycin has been linked with colonisation with organisms such as VRE [72]. Literature regarding subsequent colonisation of patients with VRE after exposure to vancomycin surgical antimicrobial prophylaxis is conflicting; in a study by Merrer et al., use of vancomycin surgical antimicrobial prophylaxis was not associated with subsequent VRE colonisation [73]. In contrast, Kachroo et al. demonstrated a 4% incidence of VRE colonisation after vancomycin surgical antimicrobial prophylaxis, but the authors did not provide data on the prevalence of VRE within their centre; therefore, establishing a causal link is challenging [71]. Thus, further research is required to assess the risks and benefits for the prevention of methicillin-resistant staphylococcal infections.

Another area of current debate is the role of extended prophylaxis coverage for Gram-negative bacilli. In a before and after study, the incidence of surgical site infection following the addition of weight-based dosing of gentamicin to cefazolin in patients undergoing hip arthroplasty was examined. The study group includes 4122 hip arthroplasties receiving cefazolin and 1267 hip arthroplasties receiving cefazolin plus gentamicin. In parallel, the researchers also include 4695 knee arthroplasties receiving cefazolin throughout both time periods as a quasi-'control' group, presumably as an attempt to account for secular trends. With the inclusion of gentamicin prophylaxis, the incidence of surgical site infections decreased from 1.19% to 0.56% (Fisher's exact test $P = 0.05$). Of note, the rate of infections due to Gram-negative bacilli decreased from 0.32% to 0% ($P = 0.048$) [74]. There was no increase in toxicities associated with aminoglycoside therapy [75].

Finally, there is ongoing concern about the association between cephalosporin use, including as surgical antimicrobial prophylaxis, and *Clostridium difficile* infections [76]. Earlier research of 108 participants receiving a single dose of cephalosporin as prophylaxis observed a high proportion of patients with *C. difficile* detected on subsequent faecal samples [77]. Following a single dose of cefazolin, 14.3% of patients had toxin-positive *C. difficile* detected; of note, however, no patient had symptomatic disease [77].

In response to concerns about increasing rates of *C. difficile* infections, the antibiotic regimen at many Scottish hospitals was altered as part of a broader policy to limit cephalosporin use [78]. Bell and colleagues examined the effect on preoperative acute kidney injury following the change in surgical antimicrobial prophylaxis protocols from cefuroxime to flucloxacillin and gentamicin for total joint replacement surgery. In this large cohort study ($n = 12,482$) applying time-series analysis methodology, the alteration of the surgical antimicrobial prophylaxis regimen to flucloxacillin and gentamicin was associated with 94% increase (95% CI 93.8–94.3%) in the incidence of acute kidney injury in patients undergoing orthopaedic procedures (excluding patients that had surgery for fractured neck of femur, in whom co-amoxiclav was given as prophylaxis) [78]. This increased incidence of acute kidney injury was also noted to have a higher mortality rate within the first year of surgery (20.8% vs 8.2%) [78]. The authors also noted *C. difficile* rates fell in all patients including those undergoing repairs for a fracture neck of femur (who received co-amoxiclav); therefore, the authors suggested that factors other than the prophylaxis might be driving the development of *C. difficile* infections [78]. Consequently, such findings led to a change back to the original prescribing policies [78].

Overall, the current literature including general expert consensus and guidelines still recommends a first- or second-generation cephalosporin such as cefazolin and cefuroxime, respectively, to cover the most common pathogens [55]. Current recommendations regarding vancomycin therapy suggest its use should be reserved for patients with documented immediate hypersensitivity to beta-lactams and those with known methicillin-resistant *S. aureus* colonisation [55].

Route and Dose   The accepted route for antimicrobial prophylaxis in joint replacement surgery is intravenous. It is also common practice for antibiotic-loaded cement to be used in addition to systemic antimicrobials in many centres (the use of antibiotic-loaded cement is discussed in detail in the section below).

One group has investigated intraosseous administration of vancomycin in a small ($n = 30$), poor-quality randomised controlled trial that was not powered to assess clinical outcomes [79]. There are limited data to support alternative routes of administration, and intravenous administration of surgical antimicrobial prophylaxis remains the standard method of administration [55].

Systematic reviews regarding surgical antimicrobial prophylaxis in joint replacement surgery do not specify the optimal dose of any particular antimicrobial agent [56, 58]. First- and second-generation cephalosporins are relatively comparable in terms of pharmacokinetics [80–82]. Early research suggested that cefazolin exhibited greater bone concentrations than that of cephalothin and cephradine: of note, a dose of 1-gram cephalothin did not reach sufficient levels in the bone to have activity against *S. aureus* [81]. Similarly, Williams et al. compared 152 assays of serum and bone concentrations of five cephalosporins (dosed at either 1 or 2 g), cephalothin, cefazolin, cefamandole, cefoxitin and ceforanide, from 95 patients undergoing hip or knee replacement surgery [82]. The antibiotics had reasonable serum and bone levels with activity against the most commonly isolated pathogens. However, as with the earlier study, cephalothin had the lowest detected levels in bone [82]. Based upon the comparable efficacy and the low cost of cefazolin, the authors recommended intravenous cefazolin 2 g preoperatively for joint replacement surgery [82].

Moine and Fish attempted to define optimal dosing using Monte Carlo simulation to examine the pharmacokinetics and pharmacodynamics of seven antimicrobials in colorectal patients [83]. The study included a comparison of 1- or 2-g of cefazolin, examining its activity against a range of microorganisms including *S. aureus* and *Escherichia coli* [83]. The authors applied susceptibility breakpoints recommended by the Clinical and Laboratory Standards Institute (CLSI) for cefazolin of 1 mg/L for *E. coli* and 8 mg/L for *S. aureus* [84]. The probability of target attainment was computed to assess the probability that the drug concentration exceeded the minimum inhibitory concentration of the organism studied [83]. When examining the activity against *E. coli*, both a 1-g and 2-g dose of cefazolin had a probability of target attainment of 100% out to 4 h post dose. In contrast with *S. aureus*, the probability of target attainment with 1-g cefazolin rapidly decreased to 0% 4 h post dose. A dose of 2-g cefazolin maintained a probability of target attainment above 90% throughout the time period [83]. The authors therefore recommended that, if cefazolin were used, higher doses (2 g) should be used for surgical antimicrobial prophylaxis [83]. Of note, this study used population data from nonobese patients [83].

There are limited studies examining cefazolin pharmaco-kinetics in obese patients undergoing arthroplasty. This has been examined in bariatric surgery, with conflicting results. A study by Brill et al., using microdialysis techniques, demonstrated reduced adipose tissue levels with 2 g of cefazolin in eight morbidly obese patients (body mass index > 40 kg/m^2) compared to seven nonobese patients [85]. Applying Monte Carlo simulation techniques, the probability of attaining an antibiotic level above 4 mg/L in the subcutaneous tissue decreased over time in the morbidly obese population to a probability of 66.3% compared to 94.9% in the nonobese population 4 h after the initial dose of cefazolin [85]. The authors concluded that dose adjustment was required in the morbidly obese population but did not recommend whether the dose should be increased or whether the dosing interval should be shorter [85]. This contrasts to the conclusions by Chen et al. [86]. As with the study by Brill et al., this study was undertaken in a cohort of morbidly obese patients undergoing bariatric surgery (mean body mass index = 46 ± 8 kg/m^2). High pressure liquid chromatography assays were used to measure cefazolin concentrations in blood and subcutaneous adipose tissue [86]. The authors noted that the cefazolin concentrations 'exceeded 1 mg/L in virtually all samples' without reporting the exact percentage nor the percentage of patients with cefazolin levels above 4 mg/L [86]. In addition, there were no operations extending beyond 4 h, with mean surgical times of less than 3 h [86]. The difference in methodology and operation length could account for the different findings and conclusions drawn [85, 86].

In an attempt to examine the clinical impact of surgical antimicrobial prophylaxis dosing in obesity, Ho and colleagues conducted research comparing dosing regimen of cefazolin for surgical prophylaxis in morbidly obese patients. The study included patients classified as morbidly obese (body mass index 40–50 kg/m^2: n = 15) and super obese (body mass index > 50 kg/m^2: n = 10) [87]. A subset of the study compared 2 g with 3 g of cefazolin in the super obese group with no difference observed in the mean concentration nor time above the minimum inhibitory concentration (defined as 8 mcg/mL) [87]. The authors concluded 2 g of cefazolin provides sufficient coverage for most general surgical procedures regardless of the patient's body mass index [87].

A further retrospective study compared 99 obese (body mass index $\geq$30 kg/m^2) and 96 nonobese (body mass index <30 kg/m^2) patients who received 2 g of cefazolin preoperatively in a range of surgical procedures [88]. There was no difference in the number of infections between obese and nonobese patients in this small study (five versus seven, respectively; P = 0.56) [88]. Similarly, a retrospective cohort study of 335 pregnant women undergoing caesarean delivery compared the efficacy of preoperative cefazolin 2 g with 3 g. There was no significant difference in surgical site infection rates between the 2-g and 3-g cefazolin cohorts (13.1% for both cohorts; P = 0.996; adjusted OR 1.33, 0.64–2.74). Therefore, current literature has not suggested evidence to support increased doses of cefazolin in obesity: despite this, guidelines have included recommendations to increase cefazolin dosing to 3 g for patients weighing >120 kg [55]. This recommendation was made in recognition of the paucity of evidence and reflected expert consensus that, given the association of obesity and surgical site infections, coupled with the tolerability and low cost of cefazolin, this increased dose was justifiable [55].

Given the concerns regarding cephalosporin exposure and risk of *Clostridium difficile* infection, recent studies have also examined the pharmacokinetics of alternate regimens [78]. Torkington et al. investigated the bone penetration of intravenous flucloxacillin (2 g) and gentamicin (3 mg/kg ideal body weight) in hip and knee arthroplasty. A sample of 40 participants demonstrated differing concentrations between knees and hips, with higher concentrations of both antimicrobials observed in hips [89]. The authors postulated that this observed difference may be due to the use of a tourniquet in knee arthroplasties [89]. Overall, gentamicin had subtherapeutic levels against *S. epidermidis* in most knee arthroplasties; however, the authors concluded that when used in combination with flucloxacillin, this regimen provided effective cover of *S. aureus* and *S. epidermidis* in 97.5% of patients [89].

The current literature, while low in evidence quality, supports the administration of 2-g cefazolin intravenously, with consideration of increasing the dose to 3 g in patients weighing >120 kg [55].

Timing of Administration   Meta-analysis of 13 observational studies conducted in the recent WHO recommendations demonstrated administration of surgical antimicrobial prophylaxis after skin incision was associated with a significantly higher risk of surgical site infection (OR 1.89; 95% CI 1.05–3.4) [7]. Administration of surgical antimicrobial prophylaxis greater than 120 min before skin incision also was associated with an increased risk of infection (OR 5.26; 95% CI 3.29–8.39) [7]. The WHO recommended that antimicrobials with a short half-life (such as cefazolin) be administered within 60 min prior to skin incision; however, it was noted that there was limited supporting data for this recommendation [7]. Subsequent to the publication of these guidelines, a large randomised controlled trial (n = 5580) compared 'early' (30–75 min before incision) administration of surgical antimicrobial prophylaxis with 1.5 g of cefuroxime with 'late' administration (0–30 min before incision) of the same antimicrobial and included a range of surgical procedures including orthopaedic surgery [90]. Patients were followed for 30 days post operation, and surgical site infections were defined in accordance with the CDC definitions [90]. There was a 13–14% crossover rate between the two study arms observed; in addition, 0.9% of the patients assigned to the late arm received prophylactic antimicrobials after incision [90]. The median time to administration of antimicrobials was 42 min (interquartile range 30–55) in the early arm and 16 min (interquartile range 10–25) in the late arm [90]. The incidence of surgical site infection was 5% in both arms (OR 0.93; 95% CI 0.72–1.21). It was noted that the study was powered to detect a larger effect size, influencing interpretation [90]. The authors concluded that there was insufficient evidence that recommends an optimal time window for surgical antimicrobial prophylaxis [90].

In relation to total knee joint replacement, the timing of surgical antimicrobial prophylaxis is also influenced by tourniquet application. Inflation of the tourniquet reduces blood supply to the operative field and may influence the antimicrobial concentrations present in the tissues [91, 92]. Therefore, surgical antimicrobial prophylaxis should be administered to ensure peak concentrations are achieved prior to this point to ensure efficacy [55, 92]. Early literature suggested the tourniquet inflation should occur 5–10 min after the administration of surgical antimicrobial prophylaxis [91, 93, 94].

Contrary to these recommendations, Soriano et al. conducted a randomised double-blind placebo-controlled, superiority trial comparing administration of 1.5-g cefuroxime either 10–30 min prior to tourniquet inflation or 10 min prior to tourniquet release in patients undergoing primary knee arthroplasty [92]. The study enrolled 908 patients and 28 patients (3.1%) developed a prosthetic joint infection after 12-month follow-up [92]. There was no difference in the incidence of infection between the two arms (3.6% in the standard arm versus 2.6%; $P = 0.44$). The authors acknowledged that the study was potentially underpowered [92]. Therefore, it is difficult to draw definitive conclusions from this study.

Overall, the literature regarding specific, optimal surgical antimicrobial timing is inconclusive. Current WHO recommendations suggest within 120 min prior to incision; however, practical considerations such as the pharmacokinetics of the antimicrobial will influence this, and therefore shorter-acting antimicrobial such as cefazolin theoretically should be administered within 60 min [7, 55, 90].

Intraoperative Redosing A repeat intraoperative dose is required if the procedure exceeds two half-lives of the antimicrobial from the time of administration or if there is excessive blood loss during the procedure [55]. The half-life for cefazolin is 1.2–2.2 h in adults with normal renal function: therefore, the recommended interval for redosing cefazolin is 4 h [55]. Again, the evidence behind such recommendations is limited in terms of small sample sizes and lack of significance. Swoboda and colleagues compared the effect of intraoperative blood loss on serum and tissue concentrations for both cefazolin (1 g) and gentamicin (1.8 mg/kg) in eleven patients who underwent elective spinal procedures [95]. The concentration of cefazolin measured 1 h following administration, correlated with the estimated blood loss ($r = 0.73$; $P = 0.04$): this observation was more pronounced with gentamicin ($r = 0.82$; $P = 0.01$) [95]. Based upon the pharmacokinetic values measured, the authors proposed that additional doses of cefazolin be administered when the operation duration exceeded 4 h or if blood loss exceeded 1500 mL [95].

Duration With respect to the optimal duration of prophylaxis, a single dose at the time of surgery appears to be as effective as multiple preoperative courses. In a retrospective cohort study by Tang et al., cefazolin as a single dose had a similar efficacy to three doses of cefuroxime in a prospective cohort of 1367 knee and hip arthroplasties [96]. An earlier randomised controlled trial by Mauerhan et al. of 1354 patients also found no difference in infection incidence between those who received a 24-h regimen of intravenous cefuroxime and those who received a 3-day regimen of cefazolin after 12-month follow-up (2.9% and 3.3%, respectively; 95% CI -2.0–2.1%; $P = 0.94$) [97]. Similarly, Wymenga et al. compared the efficacy of one dose of cefuroxime to three doses in 2651 hip or knee arthroplasties [98]. This randomised controlled trial was designed to assess superiority and applied a one-sided chi-squared test. Overall, the incidence of prosthetic joint infection after 12-month follow-up was 0.83% in the one-dose group compared with 0.45% in the three-dose group (chi-squared [one sided] $P = 0.17$) [98].

Interestingly, taking into account the null finding, the authors concluded that the three-dose regimen was recommended pending further research [98].

The recent WHO guidelines strongly recommended against prolonged surgical antimicrobial prophylaxis [7]. A meta-analysis of 69 randomised controlled trials found no difference in surgical site infections incidence with a single dose of prophylaxis at the time of incision versus continuing prophylaxis in the postoperative period (OR 0.89; 95% CI 0.77–1.03) [7]. Large cohort studies have also demonstrated that prolongation of prophylaxis is associated with increased risk of *C. difficile* infection and surgical site infections due to antimicrobial-resistant bacteria [79, 99–101]. In orthopaedic procedures, current evidence suggests a single dose of antimicrobial prophylaxis is sufficient and further doses are not warranted [55].

5.3.6   Antimicrobial-Loaded Cement

The use of antibiotic-loaded cement for fixation of the prosthesis is a common practice in joint replacement surgery. The Norwegian Arthroplasty Register recently published data from 56,275 cemented and uncemented primary hip replacements [102]. Overall, 63% of total hip joint replacements had antibiotic-loaded cement, 28% had cement without antibiotics, and 9% of hip replacement surgeries were uncemented. The RR of revision for infection was higher in replacements without antibiotic-loaded cement compared to operations where antibiotic-loaded cement was used (RR 1.5; 95% CI 1.1–2.0). There was no difference in risk of revision for infection between uncemented hip replacements and antibiotic-loaded cemented replacements (RR 1.2; 95% CI 0.7–2.0) [102]. In earlier analysis by this same research group, the efficacy of antibiotic-loaded cement appeared to be additive to the use of systemic antimicrobial prophylaxis: the risk of revision for infection was almost twofold higher when systemic prophylactic antibiotics were used in isolation, compared to the combined use of systemic prophylactic antibiotics and antibiotic-impregnated cement (RR 1.8; 95% CI 1.1–3.0) [103].

Of importance, in the updated study, the authors noted marked change in practice over the 16-year observation period. The majority of surgeries without antibiotic-loaded cement were performed before 1995; after that period, there was a steep decline in the frequency of surgeries performed without antibiotic-loaded cement. When examining the data after 1995, no difference between groups was observed [102]. A time series analysis was not performed, and there was no adjustment for changes in infection prevention or surgical techniques, including different antibiotic-loaded cement products, which may impact the risk of surgical site infection [102, 104].

The benefit of antibiotic-loaded cement in total knee joint replacement surgery has also been examined. A study by Bohm et al., using data from the Canadian Joint Replacement Registry and the Hospital Morbidity Database over a 5-year period (2003–2008), examined the impact of antibiotic-loaded cement on revision rates in 29,016 knee replacement surgeries [105]. There was no difference in the risk of revision in the antibiotic-loaded cement compared to cement without antibiotic, but, as noted by the authors, the outcome examined was risk for revision overall, not revision specifically for infection [105]. This is a crude marker for infection and therefore definitive evidence to support antibiotic-loaded cement in total knee replacement is lacking.

The meta-analysis performed by Berríos-Torres et al. identified two randomised controlled trials, both at moderate risk of bias, which demonstrated a reduced risk of deep surgical site infections when cefuroxime was incorporated into the cement (OR 0.08; 95% CI 0.01–0.59); however, the authors concluded that 'available evidence suggests uncertain trade-offs between the benefits and harms regarding cement modifications and the prevention of biofilm formation or surgical site infections in prosthetic joint arthroplasty' and no recommendation was provided [5].

Of note, the majority of antibiotic-loaded cement contains an aminoglycoside antibiotic [104]. Extrapolation of the benefit with different classes of antimicrobials is problematic. In addition to lack of clarity regarding the efficacy of antibiotic-loaded cement, there are a number of concerns. The cost-effectiveness of this practice has not been established. This question was examined by Cummins et al. who applied Markov decision analysis to model the cost-utility of antibiotic-loaded cement for primary joint replacement surgery [106]. Overall, the model demonstrated that the use of antibiotic-loaded cement was associated with a decrease in costs of US$200 per patient; however, the model was sensitive to changes in costs of the procedure and patient age [106]. Similarly, in the study by Gutowski et al., examining the use of the premixed tobramycin cement, the estimated cost was US$112,606.67 per case of prosthetic joint infection prevented [107].

In addition, the downstream consequences of antimicrobial use including allergic reactions, toxicity and the emergence of antimicrobial resistance require consideration. Lutro et al. examined the changing susceptibility of microorganisms isolated from prosthetic joint infections over time using data from the Norwegian Joint Replacement Registry and observed an increasing rate of aminoglycoside resistance from 47% in 1993–1997 to 68% in 2003–2007 [59]. The increasing use of aminoglycoside antibiotic-loaded cement was postulated as a potential explanation for this observation [59]. Despite these concerns, use of antibiotic-loaded cement in primary joint replacement is an embedded practice [11].

5.3.7   Antiseptic Irrigation

In addition to skin antisepsis, antiseptic irrigation of the surgical wound is frequently performed prior to closure to kill any organisms that have contaminated the wound during surgery. In the CDC guidelines, this issue was specifically examined in a meta-analysis [5]. Two randomised controlled trials in clean spinal surgery of moderate quality were identified comparing dilute povidone-iodine solution with normal saline. This analysis demonstrated a reduced incidence of deep surgical site infections (OR 0.08; 95% CI 0.01–0.58) [5]. There did not appear to be an increase in the risk of adverse events or wound healing reported. Two included randomised controlled trials reported increased levels of free iodine observed; however, there were no reports of toxicity [5]. The authors of the guidelines concluded that there were 'uncertain trade-offs between the benefits and harms', but they included a weak recommendation for consideration to irrigate wounds with dilute aqueous iodophor solutions [5].

5.3.8   Wound Closure

The method of wound closure may also impact on the risk of developing prosthetic joint infections. In an early meta-analysis by Smith et al. including six studies, the use of staples was associated with an increased risk of infections (RR 3.83; 95% CI 1.38–10.68) [108]. The authors noted that the evidence was predominantly derived from hip arthroplasty cohorts, in addition to significant methodological issues [108]. A subsequent meta-analysis by Krishnan et al. identified a further seven studies in addition to the six studies identified by Smith et al. in orthopaedic surgery (predominantly lower limb surgery) [109]. In this analysis, there was no difference in infections between the two wound closure methods (RR 1.06; 95% CI 0.46–2.44). There was no difference observed on subgroup analysis with hip or with knee arthroplasties [109]. Both authors concluded that further, well-executed randomised controlled trials were required [108, 109].

5.3.9   Operating Theatre Airflow and Space Suits

The role of clean air technology in the prevention of prosthetic joint infection is controversial. An early randomised controlled trial in hip and knee arthroplasty by Lidwell et al. comparing traditional (turbulent) to ultraclean airflow (laminar) demonstrated a significant reduction in the incidence of infection with the use of ultraclean air from 1.5% to 0.6%, respectively (RR 2.6; 95% CI 1.6–4.2) [110]. One criticism of this study is that prophylactic antibiotics were not used in 28% of cases and the use was not controlled; on subgroup analysis, the absence of surgical antimicrobial prophylaxis was associated with a fourfold increase risk of infection (RR 4.0; 95% CI 2.6–6.2) [110]. The authors acknowledged that this may be a potential source of bias [110]. Subsequent studies have not replicated these findings. Indeed, Salvati et al. observed an increased rate of infections in knee arthroplasty conducted in laminar airflow operation suites. The authors hypothesised that the position of theatre personnel with regard to the patient and direction of air flow may be associated with potential bacterial contamination of the wound [111]. A recent meta-analysis by Bischoff et al. compared laminar with conventional turbulent ventilation in a number of procedure types, predominantly incorporating data from large registry-based cohort studies [112]. The authors identified eight cohort studies in hip replacement surgery including 330,146 patients and did not demonstrate evidence to support use of laminar over conventional airflow (OR 1.29; 95% CI 0.98–1.71). When analysing six cohort studies in total knee joint replacement surgery ($n = 134,368$ patients), there was no observed difference between airflow systems (OR 1.08; 95% CI 0.77–1.52) [112]. Similarly, the authors of the WHO guideline recommended against the use of laminar airflow ventilation systems as a conditional recommendation based on 'low to very low quality of evidence' [7].

Berríos-Torres et al. also investigated the role of 'body exhaust' or 'space suits' commonly worn by orthopaedic surgeons. Data was extracted from three observational studies, using a range of case definitions for infection including deep infections requiring reoperation, infections requiring revision or clinical diagnosis of infection [5]. There was limited data to support the use of space suits. Indeed, a large registry study by Hooper et al., included in the meta-analysis, demonstrated a significant increase in the risk of revision surgery for infection when space suits were used [113].

In a cost-effectiveness analysis by Graves et al., comparing the risk of surgical site infections following total hip arthroplasty with or without laminar flow, there was no difference in the risk of infection (OR 1.96; 95% CI 0.52–5.37) in patients that received systemic and cement impregnated antimicrobials [114]. Similarly, there was no benefit with the use of space suits in conventional airflow theatres (OR 3.72; 95% CI 0.38–13.75) or laminar airflow (OR 5.00, 95% CI 0.73–16.87) [114]. The authors noted that the use of laminar flow or laminar flow with space suits increased annual costs by £5,032,528 and £9,106,352, respectively, with poorer health outcomes in NHS hospitals compared with the conventional airflow theatres when controlling for antimicrobial use [114]. The authors concluded that consideration by healthcare authorities and providers should be given to divest these practices [114].

5.4   Postoperative

In addition to the specific topics addressed below, strategies in the postoperative period to reduce the risk of prosthetic joint infection include general attention to hand hygiene and expeditious removal of intravenous access and other devices, such as indwelling urinary catheters [115].

5.4.1   Wound Care

Research has focused on a number of aspects of wound care for prevention of surgical site infections in the preoperative period. Different dressing types have been examined, but there is no evidence to support one form of wound dressing compared to another for prevention of surgical site infections [116]. Drain tubes are frequently used in orthopaedic surgery in order to minimise haematoma formation. A Cochrane review was conducted by Parker et al., examining the impact of closed suction drainage of orthopaedic surgical wounds. When examining the impact of drainage on all wound infections in 30 studies

(n = 5370), the use of closed suction drainage of wounds was not associated with a reduction in wound infection (RR 0.84; 95% CI 0.61, 1.15), and there was no observed difference when analysed according to joint type or for prevention of prosthetic joint infection [117]. Interestingly, the use of closed suction drainage also did not impact on the risk of haematoma (RR 0.78; 95% CI 0.52–1.17) [117]. Similarly, a second Cochrane review by Toon et al. did not show a difference with early (within 48 h) or delayed removal of dressings following surgery [118].

5.4.2   Blood Transfusion

An association between prosthetic joint infection and blood transfusion has been noted in a number of studies [23]. It is difficult to delineate whether the increased risk relates to the blood transfusion itself, increased complexity of surgery and other perioperative medical complications such as acute myocardial infarction or higher rates of bleeding and haematoma at the surgical site [10, 23]. In the CDC guidelines, the role of transfusion in arthroplasty was examined in a number of meta-analyses. Comparing transfusion or no transfusion, data from six studies, including two randomised controlled trials, demonstrated an increased risk of surgical site infections (OR 1.56; 95% CI 1.18–2.06), but this risk was not observed when only the data from randomised controlled trials were analysed (OR 1.07; 95% CI 0.39–2.89) [5]. On further analysis, it appeared that revision surgeries were more likely to require blood transfusions compared with primary arthroplasty, suggesting that transfusion may plausibly be the result of more complicated surgery [5]. The guideline authors did not provide specific recommendations regarding blood transfusions in this setting, only providing the comment that blood transfusions should not be withheld as a strategy to prevent prosthetic joint infections [5].

5.4.3 Anticoagulation

Linked with the issues of wound drainage, haematoma formation and blood transfusion, the use of anticoagulation in the preoperative setting was also examined by Berríos-Torres et al. The authors compared different anticoagulant agents, different anticoagulant strategies and different timings of institution of venous thromboembolism prophylaxis without demonstrating any benefit of one approach over another [5]. Overall this was considered an unresolved issue [5].

5.4.4 Prophylaxis with Dental Procedures

There has been long-standing clinical concern about the risk of haematogenous seeding of the prosthetic joint following dental procedures with disparate views on the role of antimicrobial prophylaxis in this setting. The estimated risk of haematogenous seeding of a prosthetic joint is extremely low, estimated at 0.00023 (range, 0.00012–0.00034) per dental visit [119]. In 2014, the American Dental Association Council undertook as systematic review as part of the update of their guidelines for antimicrobial prophylaxis for dental procedures in patients with a prosthetic joint [120]. The panel included data from four case-control studies examining if an association existed between dental procedures and subsequent prosthetic joint infection [120]. There were limitations identified in the studies included; however, based on the review, the panel recommended against the use of prophylactic antimicrobial prior to dental procedures with moderate certainty. The authors highlighted the lack of clear data demonstrating a causal link between dental procedures and prosthetic joint infection in addition to the potential unintended harms for widespread antimicrobial exposure. In a cited study, Lockhart et al. estimated the potential amount and cost of antimicrobial prophylaxis if prophylaxis was administered for dental procedures in patients with prosthetic joints [121]. The authors estimated that this would potentially lead to 2,979,714–11,918,854 antimicrobial prescriptions with a cost of

US $12,008,245–48,032,982 annually based on data and cost estimates in 2010 [121]. A Markov model developed by Skaar et al. examining the cost-effectiveness of prophylaxis in this setting demonstrated that avoidance of dental prophylaxis was the most cost-effective strategy [119]. The administration of prophylaxis was associated with increased costs, with no incremental increase in quality-adjusted life years (QALY) [119].

References

1. Kurtz SM, Ong KL, Lau E, Bozic KJ. Impact of the economic downturn on total joint replacement demand in the United States: updated projections to 2021. J Bone Joint Surg Am. 2014;96(8):624–30.
2. Australian Orthopaedic Association. National Joint Replacement Registry (website) Adelaide. https://aoanjrr.dmac.adelaide.edu.au/. Accessed 21 June 2017.
3. Kurtz SM, Lau E, Schmier J, Ong KL, Zhao K, Parvizi J. Infection burden for hip and knee arthroplasty in the United States. J Arthroplast. 2008;23(7):984–91.
4. Umscheid CA, Mitchell MD, Doshi JA, Agarwal R, Williams K, Brennan PJ. Estimating the proportion of healthcare-associated infections that are reasonably preventable and the related mortality and costs. Infect Control Hosp Epidemiol. 2011;32(2):101–14.
5. Berríos-Torres SI, Umscheid CA, Bratzler DW, Leas B, Stone EC, Kelz RR, Healthcare Infection Control Practices Advisory Committee, et al. Centers for disease control and prevention guideline for the prevention of surgical site infection. JAMA Surg. 2017. https://doi.org/10.1001/jamasurg.2017.0904. [Epub ahead of print].
6. Allegranzi B, Zayed B, Bischoff P, Kubilay NZ, de Jonge S, de Vries F, et al. New WHO recommendations on intraoperative and postoperative measures for surgical site infection prevention: an evidence-based global perspective. Lancet Infect Dis. 2016;16(12):e288–303.
7. Allegranzi B, Bischoff P, de Jonge S, Kubilay NZ, Zayed B, Gomes SM, et al. New WHO recommendations on preoperative measures for surgical site infection prevention:

an evidence-based global perspective. Lancet Infect Dis. 2016;16(12):e276–e87.

8. Mangram AJ, Horan TC, Pearson ML, Silver LC, Jarvis WR. Guideline for prevention of surgical site infection, 1999. Hospital Infection Control Practices Advisory Committee. Infect Control Hosp Epidemiol. 1999;20(4):250–78. quiz 79–80.

9. Bratzler DW, Houck PM. Antimicrobial prophylaxis for surgery: an advisory statement from the National Surgical Infection Prevention Project. Am J Surg. 2005;189(4):395–404.

10. Peel TN, Dowsey MM, Daffy JR, Stanley PA, Choong PF, Buising KL. Risk factors for prosthetic hip and knee infections according to arthroplasty site. J Hosp Infect. 2011;79(2):129–33.

11. Parvizi J, Gehrke T, Musculoskeletal Infection Society. Proceedings of the international consensus on periprosthetic joint infection. 2013. http://www.msis-na.org/wp-content/themes/msis-temp/pdf/ism-periprosthetic-joint-information.pdf. Accessed 21 June 2017.

12. Kluytmans J, van Belkum A, Verbrugh H. Nasal carriage of *Staphylococcus aureus*: epidemiology, underlying mechanisms, and associated risks. Clin Microbiol Rev. 1997;10(3):505–20.

13. Gorwitz RJ, Kruszon-Moran D, McAllister SK, McQuillan G, McDougal LK, Fosheim GE, et al. Changes in the prevalence of nasal colonization with *Staphylococcus aureus* in the United States, 2001-2004. J Infect Dis. 2008;197(9):1226–34.

14. Hacek DM, Robb WJ, Paule SM, Kudrna JC, Stamos VP, Peterson LR. *Staphylococcus aureus* nasal decolonization in joint replacement surgery reduces infection. Clin Orthop Relat Res. 2008;466(6):1349–55.

15. Kalmeijer MD, Coertjens H, van Nieuwland-Bollen PM, Bogaers-Hofman D, de Baere GJ, Stuurman A, et al. Surgical site infections in orthopedic surgery: the effect of mupirocin nasal ointment in a double-blind, randomized, placebo-controlled study. Clin Infect Dis. 2002;35(4):353–8.

16. van Rijen MM, Bonten M, Wenzel RP, Kluytmans JA. Intranasal mupirocin for reduction of *Staphylococcus aureus* infections in surgical patients with nasal carriage: a systematic review. J Antimicrob Chemother. 2008;61(2):254–61.

17. Lim MS, Marshall CL, Spelman D. Carriage of multiple subtypes of methicillin-resistant *Staphylococcus aureus* by intensive care unit patients. Infect Control Hosp Epidemiol. 2006;27(10):1063–7.

18. Young BC, Votintseva AA, Foster D, Godwin H, Miller RR, Anson LW, et al. Multi-site and nasal swabbing for carriage of *Staphylococcus aureus*: what does a single nose swab predict? J Hosp Infect. 2017;96(3):232–7.

19. Baratz MD, Hallmark R, Odum SM, Springer BD. Twenty percent of patients may remain colonized with methicillin-resistant *Staphylococcus aureus* despite a decolonization protocol in patients undergoing elective total joint arthroplasty. Clin Orthop Relat Res. 2015;473(7):2283–90.

20. Harbarth S, Fankhauser C, Schrenzel J, Christenson J, Gervaz P, Bandiera-Clerc C, et al. Universal screening for methicillin-resistant *Staphylococcus aureus* at hospital admission and nosocomial infection in surgical patients. JAMA. 2008;299(10):1149–57.

21. Hayden MK, Lolans K, Haffenreffer K, Avery TR, Kleinman K, Li H, et al. Chlorhexidine and mupirocin susceptibility of methicillin-resistant *Staphylococcus aureus* isolates in the REDUCE-MRSA trial. J Clin Microbiol. 2016;54(11):2735–42.

22. Walsh EE, Greene L, Kirshner R. Sustained reduction in methicillin-resistant *staphylococcus aureus* wound infections after cardiothoracic surgery. Arch Intern Med. 2011;171(1):68–73.

23. Pulido L, Ghanem E, Joshi A, Purtill JJ, Parvizi J, Pulido L, et al. Periprosthetic joint infection: the incidence, timing, and predisposing factors. Clin Orthop Relat Res. 2008;466(7):1710–5.

24. Wilson MG, Kelley K, Thornhill TS. Infection as a complication of total knee-replacement arthroplasty. Risk factors and treatment in sixty-seven cases. J Bone Joint Surg Am. 1990;72-A(6):878–83.

25. Surin VV, Sundholm K, Backman L. Infection after total hip replacement. J Bone Joint Surg (Br). 1983;65-Br(4):412–8.

26. Sousa R, Munoz-Mahamud E, Quayle J, Dias da Costa L, Casals C, Scott P, et al. Is asymptomatic bacteriuria a risk factor for prosthetic joint infection? Clin Infect Dis. 2014;59(1):41–7.

27. Cordero-Ampuero J, Gonzalez-Fernandez E, Martinez-Velez D, Esteban J. Are antibiotics necessary in hip arthroplasty with asymptomatic bacteriuria? Seeding risk with/without treatment. Clin Orthop Relat Res. 2013;471(12):3822–9.

28. Lawrence VA, Gafni A, Gross M. The unproven utility of the preoperative urinalysis: economic evaluation. J Clin Epidemiol. 1989;42(12):1185–92.

29. Webster J, Osborne S. Preoperative bathing or showering with skin antiseptics to prevent surgical site infection. Cochrane Database Syst Rev. 2015;2:Cd004985.

30. Johnson AJ, Daley JA, Zywiel MG, Delanois RE, Mont MA. Preoperative chlorhexidine preparation and the incidence of surgical site infections after hip arthroplasty. J Arthroplast. 2010;25(6 Suppl):98–102.

31. Karki S, Cheng AC. Impact of non-rinse skin cleansing with chlorhexidine gluconate on prevention of healthcare-associated infections and colonization with multi-resistant organisms: a systematic review. J Hosp Infect. 2012;82(2):71–84.

32. Zywiel M, Daley J, Delanois R, Naziri Q, Johnson A, Mont M. Advance pre-operative chlorhexidine reduces the incidence of surgical site infections in knee arthroplasty. Int Orthop. 2011;35(7):1001–6.

33. Eiselt D. Presurgical skin preparation with a novel 2% chlorhexidine gluconate cloth reduces rates of surgical site infection in orthopaedic surgical patients. Orthop Nurs. 2009;28(3):141–5.

34. Tanner J, Norrie P, Melen K. Preoperative hair removal to reduce surgical site infection. Cochrane Database Syst Rev. 2011;11:CD004122.

35. Alexander JW, Fischer JE, Boyajian M, Palmquist J, Morris MJ. The influence of hair-removal methods on wound infections. Arch Surg. 1983;118(3):347–52.

36. Tanner J, Dumville JC, Norman G, Fortnam M. Surgical hand antisepsis to reduce surgical site infection. Cochrane Database Syst Rev. 2016;1:CD004288.

37. Edwards PS, Lipp A, Holmes A. Preoperative skin antiseptics for preventing surgical wound infections after clean surgery. Cochrane Database Syst Rev. 2004;3:CD003949.

38. Mangram AJ, Horan TC, Pearson ML, Silver LC, Jarvis WR. Guideline for prevention of surgical site infection, 1999. Hospital Infection Control Practices Advisory Committee. Infect Control Hosp Epidemiol. 1999;20(4):250–78.

39. Southwood RT, Rice JL, McDonald PJ, Hakendorf PH, Rozenbilds MA. Infection in experimental hip arthroplasties. J Bone Joint Surg (Br). 1985;67-Br(2):229–31.

40. Maiwald M, Chan ES. The forgotten role of alcohol: a systematic review and meta-analysis of the clinical efficacy and perceived role of chlorhexidine in skin antisepsis. PLoS One. 2012;7(9):e44277.

41. Dumville JC, McFarlane E, Edwards P, Lipp A, Holmes A, Liu Z. Preoperative skin antiseptics for preventing surgical wound

infections after clean surgery. Cochrane Database Syst Rev. 2015;4:CD003949.

42. McDonnell G, Russell AD. Antiseptics and disinfectants: activity, action, and resistance. Clin Microbiol Rev. 1999;12(1):147–79.

43. Anderson MJ, Horn ME, Lin YC, Parks PJ, Peterson ML. Efficacy of concurrent application of chlorhexidine gluconate and povidone iodine against six nosocomial pathogens. Am J Infect Control. 2010;38(10):826–31.

44. National Health and Medical Research Council Australian Guidelines for the Prevention and Control of Infection in Healthcare. Commonwealth of Australia. 2010. https://www.nhmrc.gov.au/guidelines-publications/cd33. Accessed 21 June 2017.

45. Davies BM, Patel HC. Does chlorhexidine and povidone-iodine preoperative antisepsis reduce surgical site infection in cranial neurosurgery? Ann R Coll Surg Engl. 2016;98(6):405–8.

46. Guzel A, Ozekinci T, Ozkan U, Celik Y, Ceviz A, Belen D. Evaluation of the skin flora after chlorhexidine and povidone-iodine preparation in neurosurgical practice. Surg Neurol. 2009;71(2):207–10. discussion 10.

47. Saltzman MD, Nuber GW, Gryzlo SM, Marecek GS, Koh JL. Efficacy of surgical preparation solutions in shoulder surgery. J Bone Joint Surg Am. 2009;91(8):1949–53.

48. Savage JW, Weatherford BM, Sugrue PA, Nolden MT, Liu JC, Song JK, et al. Efficacy of surgical preparation solutions in lumbar spine surgery. J Bone Joint Surg Am. 2012;94(6):490–4.

49. Lee MJ, Pottinger PS, Butler-Wu S, Bumgarner RE, Russ SM, Matsen FA 3rd. Propionibacterium persists in the skin despite standard surgical preparation. J Bone Joint Surg Am. 2014;96(17):1447–50.

50. Sabetta JR, Rana VP, Vadasdi KB, Greene RT, Cunningham JG, Miller SR, et al. Efficacy of topical benzoyl peroxide on the reduction of propionibacterium acnes during shoulder surgery. J Shoulder Elb Surg. 2015;24(7):995–1004.

51. Webster J, Alghamdi A. Use of plastic adhesive drapes during surgery for preventing surgical site infection. Cochrane Database Syst Rev. 2015;4:CD006353.

52. Falk-Brynhildsen K, Soderquist B, Friberg O, Nilsson UG. Bacterial recolonization of the skin and wound contamination during cardiac surgery: a randomized controlled trial of the use of plastic adhesive drape compared with bare skin. J Hosp Infect. 2013;84(2):151–8.

53. Falk-Brynhildsen K, Soderquist B, Friberg O, Nilsson U. Bacterial growth and wound infection following saphenous vein harvesting in cardiac surgery: a randomized controlled trial of the impact of microbial skin sealant. Eur J Clin Microbiol Infect Dis. 2014;33(11):1981–7.

54. Cordtz T, Schouenborg L, Laursen K, Daugaard HO, Buur K, Munk Christensen B, et al. The effect of incisional plastic drapes and redisinfection of operation site on wound infection following caesarean section. J Hosp Infect. 1989;13(3):267–72.

55. Bratzler DW, Dellinger EP, Olsen KM, Perl TM, Auwaerter PG, Bolon MK, et al. Clinical practice guidelines for antimicrobial prophylaxis in surgery. Am J Health Syst Pharm. 2013;70(3):195–283.

56. Voigt J, Mosier M, Darouiche R. Systematic review and meta-analysis of randomized controlled trials of antibiotics and antiseptics for preventing infection in people receiving primary total hip and knee prostheses. Antimicrob Agents Chemother. 2015;59(11):6696–707.

57. Voigt J, Mosier M, Darouiche R. Antibiotics and antiseptics for preventing infection in people receiving revision total hip and knee prostheses: a systematic review of randomized controlled trials. BMC Infect Dis. 2016;16(1):749.

58. AlBuhairan B, Hind D, Hutchinson A. Antibiotic prophylaxis for wound infections in total joint arthroplasty: a systematic review. J Bone Joint Surg (Br). 2008;90(7):915–9.

59. Lutro O, Langvatn H, Dale H, Schrama JC, Hallan G, Espehaug B, et al. Increasing resistance of coagulase-negative Staphylococci in total hip arthroplasty infections: 278 THA-revisions due to infection reported to the Norwegian Arthroplasty Register from 1993 to 2007. Adv Orthop. 2014;2014:580359.

60. Peel TN, Cheng AC, Buising KL, Choong PF. Microbiological aetiology, epidemiology, and clinical profile of prosthetic joint infections: are current antibiotic prophylaxis guidelines effective? Antimicrob Agents Chemother. 2012;56(5):2386–91.

61. Finkelstein R, Rabino G, Mashiah T, Bar-El Y, Adler Z, Kertzman V, et al. Vancomycin versus cefazolin prophylaxis for cardiac surgery in the setting of a high prevalence of methicillin-resistant staphylococcal infections. J Thorac Cardiovasc Surg. 2002;123(2):326–32.

62. Bull AL, Worth LJ, Richards MJ. Impact of vancomycin surgical antibiotic prophylaxis on the development of methicillin-sensitive *Staphylococcus aureus* surgical site infections: Report

From Australian Surveillance Data (VICNISS). Ann Surg. 2012;256(6):1089–92.

63. Saleh A, Khanna A, Chagin KM, Klika AK, Johnston D, Barsoum WK. Glycopeptides versus beta-lactams for the prevention of surgical site infections in cardiovascular and orthopedic surgery: a meta-analysis. Ann Surg. 2015;261(1):72–80.

64. Gurusamy KS, Koti R, Wilson P, Davidson BR. Antibiotic prophylaxis for the prevention of methicillin-resistant *Staphylococcus aureus* (MRSA) related complications in surgical patients. Cochrane Database Syst Rev. 2013;8:CD010268.

65. Smith EB, Wynne R, Joshi A, Liu H, Good RP. Is it time to include vancomycin for routine perioperative antibiotic prophylaxis in total joint arthroplasty patients? J Arthroplast. 2012;27(8 Suppl):55–60.

66. Ponce B, Raines BT, Reed RD, Vick C, Richman J, Hawn M. Surgical site infection after arthroplasty: comparative effectiveness of prophylactic antibiotics: do surgical care improvement project guidelines need to be updated? J Bone Joint Surg Am. 2014;96(12):970–7.

67. Liu C, Kakis A, Nichols A, Ries MD, Vail TP, Bozic KJ. Targeted use of vancomycin as perioperative prophylaxis reduces periprosthetic joint infection in revision TKA. Clin Orthop Relat Res. 2014;472(1):227–31.

68. Tornero E, Garcia-Ramiro S, Martinez-Pastor JC, Bori G, Bosch J, Morata L, et al. Prophylaxis with teicoplanin and cefuroxime reduces the rate of prosthetic joint infection after primary arthroplasty. Antimicrob Agents Chemother. 2014;59(2):831–7.

69. Sewick A, Makani A, Wu C, O'Donnell J, Baldwin KD, Lee GC. Does dual antibiotic prophylaxis better prevent surgical site infections in total joint arthroplasty? Clin Orthop Relat Res. 2012;470(10):2702–7.

70. Courtney PM, Melnic CM, Zimmer Z, Anari J, Lee G. Addition of vancomycin to cefazolin prophylaxis is associated with acute kidney injury after primary joint arthroplasty. Clin Orthop Relat Res. 2014;473(7):2197–203.

71. Kachroo S, Dao T, Zabaneh F, Reiter M, Larocco MT, Gentry LO, et al. Tolerance of vancomycin for surgical prophylaxis in patients undergoing cardiac surgery and incidence of vancomycin-resistant enterococcus colonization. Ann Pharmacother. 2006;40(3):381–5.

72. Uttley AH, Collins CH, Naidoo J, George RC. Vancomycin-resistant enterococci. Lancet. 1988;1(8575-6):57–8.

73. Merrer J, Desbouchages L, Serazin V, Razafimamonjy J, Pauthier F, Leneveu M. Comparison of routine prophylaxis with vancomycin or cefazolin for femoral neck fracture surgery: microbiological and clinical outcomes. Infect Control Hosp Epidemiol. 2006;27(12):1366–71.

74. Bosco JA, Prince Rainier RT, Catanzano AJ, Stachel AG, Phillips MS. Expanded Gram-negative antimicrobial prophylaxis reduces surgical site infections in hip arthroplasty. J Arthroplast. 2016;31(3):616–21.

75. Bosco J, Bookman J, Slover J, Edusei E, Levine B. Principles of antibiotic prophylaxis in total joint arthroplasty: current concepts. Instr Course Lect. 2016;65:467–75.

76. Yee J, Dixon CM, McLean AP, Meakins JL. Clostridium difficile disease in a department of surgery. The significance of prophylactic antibiotics. Arch Surg. 1991;126(2):241–6.

77. Privitera G, Scarpellini P, Ortisi G, Nicastro G, Nicolin R, de Lalla F. Prospective study of Clostridium difficile intestinal colonization and disease following single-dose antibiotic prophylaxis in surgery. Antimicrob Agents Chemother. 1991;35(1):208–10.

78. Bell S, Davey P, Nathwani D, Marwick C, Vadiveloo T, Sneddon J, et al. Risk of AKI with gentamicin as surgical prophylaxis. J Am Nephrol. 2014;25(11):2625–32.

79. Young SW, Zhang M, Freeman JT, Mutu-Grigg J, Pavlou P, Moore GA. The Mark Coventry award: higher tissue concentrations of vancomycin with low-dose intraosseous regional versus systemic prophylaxis in TKA: a randomized trial. Clin Orthop Relat Res. 2014;472(1):57–65.

80. Davies AJ, Lockley RM, Jones A, El-Safty M, Clothier JC. Comparative pharmacokinetics of cefamandole, cefuroxime and cephradine during total hip replacement. J Antimicrob Chemother. 1986;17(5):637–40.

81. Cunha BA, Gossling HR, Pasternak HS, Nightingale CH, Quintiliani R. The penetration characteristics of cefazolin, cephalothin, and cephradine into bone in patients undergoing total hip replacement. J Bone Joint Surg Am. 1977;59(7):856–9.

82. Williams DN, Gustilo RB, Beverly R, Kind AC. Bone and serum concentrations of five cephalosporin drugs. Relevance to prophylaxis and treatment in orthopedic surgery. Clin Orthop Relat Res. 1983;179(10):253–65.

83. Moine P, Fish DN. Pharmacodynamic modelling of intravenous antibiotic prophylaxis in elective colorectal surgery. Int J Antimicrob Agents. 2013;41(2):167–73.

84. Clinical and Laboratory Standards Institute. Methods for dilution antimicrobial susceptibility tests for bacteria that grow aerobically; Approved Standard – 9th Edition. Performance Standards for Antimicrobial Susceptibility Testing: Sixteenth Informational Supplement M07-A9 Vol. 32; No. 2. Pennsylvania, USA: CLSI; 2012.

85. Brill MJ, Houwink AP, Schmidt S, Van Dongen EP, Hazebroek EJ, van Ramshorst B, et al. Reduced subcutaneous tissue distribution of cefazolin in morbidly obese versus non-obese patients determined using clinical microdialysis. J Antimicrob Chemother. 2014;69(3):715–23.

86. Chen X, Brathwaite CE, Barkan A, Hall K, Chu G, Cherasard P, et al. Optimal cefazolin prophylactic dosing for bariatric surgery: no need for higher doses or intraoperative redosing. Obes Surg. 2017;27(3):626–9.

87. Ho VP, Nicolau DP, Dakin GF, Pomp A, Rich BS, Towe CW, et al. Cefazolin dosing for surgical prophylaxis in morbidly obese patients. Surg Infect (Larchmt). 2012;13(1):33–7.

88. Unger NR, Stein BJ. Effectiveness of pre-operative cefazolin in obese patients. Surg Infect (Larchmt). 2014;15(4):412–6.

89. Torkington MS, Davison MJ, Wheelwright EF, Jenkins PJ, Anthony I, Lovering AM, et al. Bone penetration of intravenous flucloxacillin and gentamicin as antibiotic prophylaxis during total hip and knee arthroplasty. Bone Joint J. 2017;99-b(3):358–64.

90. Weber WP, Mujagic E, Zwahlen M, Bundi M, Hoffmann H, Soysal SD, et al. Timing of surgical antimicrobial prophylaxis: a phase 3 randomised controlled trial. Lancet Infect Dis. 2017;17(6):605–14.

91. Friedman RJ, Friedrich LV, White RL, Kays MB, Brundage DM, Graham J. Antibiotic prophylaxis and tourniquet inflation in total knee arthroplasty. Clin Orthop Relat Res. 1990;260:17–23.

92. Soriano A, Bori G, Garcia-Ramiro S, Martinez-Pastor JC, Miana T, Codina C, et al. Timing of antibiotic prophylaxis for primary total knee arthroplasty performed during ischemia. Clin Infect Dis. 2008;46(7):1009–14.

93. Tomita M, Motokawa S. Effects of air tourniquet on the antibiotics concentration, in bone marrow, injected just before the start of operation. Mod Rheumatol. 2007;17(5):409–12.

94. Bannister GC, Auchincloss JM, Johnson DP, Newman JH. The timing of tourniquet application in relation to prophylactic antibiotic administration. J Bone Joint Surg (Br). 1988;70(2):322–4.

95. Swoboda SM, Merz C, Kostuik J, Trentler B, Lipsett PA. Does intraoperative blood loss affect antibiotic serum and tissue concentrations? Arch Surg. 1996;131(11):1165–72.

96. Tang WM, Chiu KY, Ng TP, Yau WP, Ching PTY, Seto WH. Efficacy of a single dose of cefazolin as a prophylactic antibiotic in primary arthroplasty. J Arthroplast. 2003; 18(6):714–8.

97. Mauerhan DR, Nelson CL, Smith DL, Fitzgerald RH Jr, Slama TG, Petty RW, et al. Prophylaxis against infection in total joint arthroplasty. One day of cefuroxime compared with three days of cefazolin. J Bone Joint Surg Am. 1994;76(1):39–45.

98. Wymenga A, van Horn J, Theeuwes A, Muytjens H, Slooff T. Cefuroxime for prevention of postoperative coxitis. One versus three doses tested in a randomized multicenter study of 2,651 arthroplasties. Acta Orthop Scand. 1992;63(1):19–24.

99. Harbarth S, Samore MH, Lichtenberg D, Carmeli Y. Prolonged antibiotic prophylaxis after cardiovascular surgery and its effect on surgical site infections and antimicrobial resistance. Circulation. 2000;101(25):2916–21.

100. Cohen SH, Gerding DN, Johnson S, Kelly CP, Loo VG, McDonald LC, et al. Clinical practice guidelines for Clostridium difficile infection in adults: 2010 update by the society for healthcare epidemiology of America (SHEA) and the infectious diseases society of America (IDSA). Infect Control Hosp Epidemiol. 2010;31(5):431–55.

101. Jobe BA, Grasley A, Deveney KE, Deveney CW, Sheppard BC. Clostridium difficile colitis: an increasing hospital-acquired illness. Am J Surg. 1995;169(5):480–3.

102. Engesaeter LB, Espehaug B, Lie SA, Furnes O, Havelin LI. Does cement increase the risk of infection in primary total hip arthroplasty? Revision rates in 56,275 cemented and uncemented primary THAs followed for 0-16 years in the Norwegian Arthroplasty Register. Acta Orthop. 2006;77(3):351–8.

103. Engesaeter LB, Lie SA, Espehaug B, Furnes O, Vollset SE, Havelin LI. Effects of antibiotic prophylaxis systemically and in bone cement on years in the Norwegian Arthroplasty Register. Acta Orthop Scand. 2003;74(6):644–51.

104. Birkeland Ø, Espehaug B, Havelin LI, Furnes O. Bone cement product and failure in total knee arthroplasty. Acta Orthop. 2017;88(1):75–81.

105. Bohm E, Zhu N, Gu J, de Guia N, Linton C, Anderson T, et al. Does adding antibiotics to cement reduce the need for

early revision in total knee arthroplasty? Clin Orthop Relat Res. 2014;472(1):162–8.

106. Cummins JS, Tomek IM, Kantor SR, Furnes O, Engesaeter LB, Finlayson SR. Cost-effectiveness of antibiotic-impregnated bone cement used in primary total hip arthroplasty. J Bone Joint Surg Am. 2009;91-A(3):634–41.

107. Gutowski CJ, Zmistowski BM, Clyde CT, Parvizi J. The economics of using prophylactic antibiotic-loaded bone cement in total knee replacement. Bone Joint J. 2014;96-b(1):65–9.

108. Smith TO, Sexton D, Mann C, Donell S. Sutures versus staples for skin closure in orthopaedic surgery: meta-analysis. Br Med J. 2010;340:c1199.

109. Krishnan R, MacNeil SD, Malvankar-Mehta MS. Comparing sutures versus staples for skin closure after orthopaedic surgery: systematic review and meta-analysis. BMJ Open. 2016;6(1):e009257.

110. Lidwell OM, Lowbury EJ, Whyte W, Blowers R, Stanley SJ, Lowe D. Effect of ultraclean air in operating rooms on deep sepsis in the joint after total hip or knee replacement: a randomised study. Br J Med. 1982;285(6334):10–4.

111. Salvati EA, Robinson RP, Zeno SM, Koslin BL, Brause BD, Wilson PD. Infection rates after 3175 total hip and total knee replacements performed with and without a horizontal unidirectional filtered air-flow system. J Bone Joint Surg Am. 1982;64-A(4):525–35.

112. Bischoff P, Kubilay NZ, Allegranzi B, Egger M, Gastmeier P. Effect of laminar airflow ventilation on surgical site infections: a systematic review and meta-analysis. Lancet Infect Dis. 2017;17(5):553–61.

113. Hooper GJ, Rothwell AG, Frampton C, Wyatt MC. Does the use of laminar flow and space suits reduce early deep infection after total hip and knee replacement?: The ten-year results of the New Zealand Joint Registry. J Bone Joint Surg (Br). 2011;93-B(1):85–90.

114. Graves N, Wloch C, Wilson J, Barnett A, Sutton A, Cooper N, et al. A cost-effectiveness modelling study of strategies to reduce risk of infection following primary hip replacement based on a systematic review. Health Technol Assess. 2016;20(54):1–144.

115. Steckelberg JM, Osmon DR. Prosthetic joint infections. In: Waldvogel FA, Bisno AL, editors. Infections associated with indwelling medical devices. 3rd ed. Washington DC: ASM; 2000. p. 173–209.

116. Dumville JC, Gray TA, Walter CJ, Sharp CA, Page T, Macefield R, et al. Dressings for the prevention of surgical site infection. Cochrane Database Syst Rev. 2016;12:CD003091.
117. Parker MJ, Livingstone V, Clifton R, McKee A. Closed suction surgical wound drainage after orthopaedic surgery. Cochrane Database Syst Rev. 2007;3:CD001825.
118. Toon CD, Lusuku C, Ramamoorthy R, Davidson BR, Gurusamy KS. Early versus delayed dressing removal after primary closure of clean and clean-contaminated surgical wounds. Cochrane Database Syst Rev. 2015;9:CD010259.
119. Skaar DD, Park T, Swiontkowski MF, Kuntz KM. Cost-effectiveness of antibiotic prophylaxis for dental patients with prosthetic joints: Comparisons of antibiotic regimens for patients with total hip arthroplasty. J Am Dent Assoc. 2015;146(11):830–9.
120. Sollecito TP, Abt E, Lockhart PB, Truelove E, Paumier TM, Tracy SL, et al. The use of prophylactic antibiotics prior to dental procedures in patients with prosthetic joints: Evidence-based clinical practice guideline for dental practitioners – a report of the American Dental Association Council on Scientific Affairs. J Am Dent Assoc. 2015;146(1):11–6.e8.
121. Lockhart PB, Blizzard J, Maslow AL, Brennan MT, Sasser H, Carew J. Drug cost implications for antibiotic prophylaxis for dental procedures. Oral Surg Oral Med Oral Pathol Oral Radiol. 2013;115(3):345–53.

Chapter 6
Prosthetic Joint Infection: Guidelines and Recommendations Update

Trisha Peel

Modern-day total joint replacement was pioneered in the 1960s for treatment of arthritis [1]. With advances in surgical technique, coupled with an ageing population, this procedure continues to grow in popularity throughout the world. US data predict that the number of hip or knee replacements will increase by over 40% from 2015 to 2020, a prediction echoed in other international studies [2–4]. Evidence supports both the clinical and cost-effectiveness of this procedure [5].

Throughout the early attempts and refinement of the procedure, infection of the prosthesis has remained a constant foe [1]. However, capturing the exact burden and risk of infection in this cohort has proven elusive. Determination of the true incidence of infection is hampered by a number of factors including the lack of uniform definition of prosthetic joint infection, lack of robust post-discharge surveillance for infection, and imprecise methods for capturing infections in

T. Peel
Department of Infectious Diseases, Monash University
and Alfred Health, Melbourne, Victoria, Australia
e-mail: trisha.peel@monash.edu

© Springer International Publishing AG 2018
T. Peel (ed.), *Prosthetic Joint Infections*,
https://doi.org/10.1007/978-3-319-65250-4_6

registries [6–8]. Overall, the accepted incidence of infection is thought to be approximately 1–3%, that is, infection of the prosthesis is an uncommon complication [9]. These infections, however, have a profound effect on patient morbidity and mortality, in addition to being a significant economic burden. Of concern, the risk of infection is increasing and is predicted to exceed 6.5% by 2030 [10].

The presence of the biofilm impacts on all aspects of diagnosis, management, and prevention of prosthetic joint infection [11]. The causative pathogens associated with prosthetic joint infection are generally skin-associated microorganisms, with a predominance of Gram-positive organisms such as coagulase-negative staphylococci. There is, however, an increasing incidence of infections due to Gram-negative bacteria observed in a number of studies [12]. Given the changing global ecology, with the emergence of antimicrobial resistance, particularly in Gram-negative bacilli, this observation is concerning and the overall impact of these organisms on elective joint replacement surgery is unknown [12].

In addition to the role of biofilm in the development of infection, patient-related factors also play a role. Given that this surgery is undertaken in older patients, comorbid diseases, such as diabetes mellitus and obesity, influence surgical outcomes. These are potentially modifiable factors; however, there are limited data to demonstrate that optimisation of these factors influences outcomes. These factors are the current focus of a number of studies.

Wound complications, including haematoma and wound ooze, have also been implicated in the development of prosthetic joint infection. Whether these wound complications are distinct entities from infection or are, in fact, early manifestations of an (as yet) undiagnosed infection remains an issue of conjecture. Furthermore, while early intervention for prolonged postoperative wound drainage is advocated, whether this intervention reduces the incidence of prosthetic joint infection is unknown [13].

In recent years, the publication of classification schemes and diagnostic criteria for prosthetic joint infection has provided a consistent framework to guide detection and management of infection. Recognition of the clinical, diagnostic, and management differences between acute and chronic infections is important. Clinical features may guide diagnosis but are imperfect; up to 15% of patients coming to revision arthroplasty with the preoperative presumptive diagnosis of aseptic failure have positive intraoperative cultures [14–16]. Development of diagnostic criteria, such as those published by the Infectious Diseases Society of America or by the Musculoskeletal Infection Society, not only aids diagnostic acumen but also to enables comparison of different tests [17, 18].

Correct differentiation between 'septic' and 'aseptic' failure remains the holy grail of research into prosthetic joint infection diagnosis. Conventional microbiology laboratory culture techniques have a low sensitivity [16]. This is further compounded by the fact that many of the common pathogens of prosthetic joint infection, such as coagulase-negative staphylococci, are also the main cause of specimen contamination.

Microbiological culture is the cornerstone of diagnosis for confirmation of infection and to assess antimicrobial susceptibility to guide treatment and preventative strategies. The likelihood of detecting infection, and differentiating infection from contamination, increases with increasing number of specimens provided [16]. In addition, collection of periprosthetic tissue samples, rather than swabs, increases yield and minimises contamination [19]. Current guidelines recommend that a minimum of three tissue specimens be obtained for microbiological culture; however, these guidelines further suggest five to six specimens is the ideal number to optimise diagnosis [16, 17].

Recent research has focused on efforts to optimise or augment laboratory techniques. This includes the application of sonication techniques, which act to release the bacteria from the biofilm attached to prostheses, thereby increasing the microbiological yield [20]. In addition, adaptation of laboratory culture methods, such as inoculation of synovial fluid and periprosthetic tissue specimens into blood culture bottles, has increased the sensitivity and accuracy of diagnosis [21–23]. Of note, when blood culture bottles for periprosthetic tissue specimen culture are used, the number of specimens required for accurate diagnosis is reduced compared with conventional techniques [24, 25].

There has also been reinvigorated interest in conventional markers such as C-reactive protein (CRP), erythrocyte sedimentation rate, and synovial fluid white cell parameters to provide more robust data on the utility of these tests. This research has provided increased clarity around diagnostic thresholds for these markers in acute and chronic settings and according to different joints [18].

In addition, new markers have been investigated, including leucocyte esterase, synovial CRP, and alpha-defensin. Initial research has suggested that these markers may be associated with improved sensitivity with preserved specificity. In particular, the early reports of alpha-defensin were particularly impressive with reported sensitivity of 97%, far in excess of conventional diagnostic tests [26]. While promising, more extensive validation of alpha-defensin is required, particularly in acute or chronic infection and in different joints. The role of these new synovial markers will be determined in the coming years. Radiology, while commonly performed, remains of uncertain utility.

Overall, given the diagnostic challenges and uncertainties, there should be a low threshold to consider infection. All patients undergoing revision surgery should have assessment of serum inflammatory markers, synovial fluid analysis, and multiple tissue samples for culture, in addition to histological examination to maximise the detection or exclusion of prosthetic joint infection.

As noted, the management of prosthetic joint infection is determined by the chronicity of infection and by the type and susceptibilities of the infecting organism(s). Neither surgery nor antibiotics administered in isolation lead to successful treatment outcomes. Therefore, a multidisciplinary approach to management with the input of both surgical and medical expertise is critical to the success of prosthetic joint infection management. In addition, understanding the effect of different antimicrobials on biofilm-associated microorganisms influences treatment outcomes.

The goals of treatment must be clearly defined to guide management decision; in particular, determining whether the goal is cure versus suppression of the infection is of import. The three broad treatment approaches are curative with prosthesis retention, curative with prosthesis removal, and infection suppression without removal of the prosthesis. Ultimately, the ideal management approach should ensure eradication of infection with preservation of a pain-free, functional joint [11].

Curative approaches with prosthetic retention can be considered in acute infections, without clinical or radiological evidence of prosthesis loosening and where the causative microorganisms are susceptible to antimicrobials with a good anti-biofilm profile [17]. Patients with chronic infection, prosthesis loosening, or infections due to microorganisms where there are no suitable anti-biofilm antimicrobial options available, and where the intent is curative, should undergo removal of the prosthesis as part of one- or two-step exchange procedures, or of joint arthrodesis [17]. Long-term suppressive antimicrobials, with retention of the prosthesis, are a reasonable management strategy in patients with significant comorbidities that would preclude more aggressive, curative approaches [17].

There have been a number of studies investigating the anti-biofilm properties of different antimicrobials both in laboratory and clinical settings. Overall, there are increasing data to support the use of rifampicin in infections with Gram-positive organisms where the intent is cure with retention of the prosthesis. The main limitation of using rifampicin is its low threshold for generation of resistance; therefore this antibiotic cannot be administered alone and must be given with a companion antimicrobial. The weight of evidence favours combination with levofloxacin as the treatment of choice for staphylococcal prosthetic joint infection. There are limited data to guide antibiotic choices for implant retention with other Gram-positive organisms. Evidence to support antimicrobial strategies for Gram-negative infections is likewise limited; however, ciprofloxacin is the accepted agent for first-line treatment [17].

Traditional recommendations for treatment for curative prosthesis retention included three months for hip and six months for knee prosthetic joint infection [11]. This was based on expert consensus. Recent research has focussed on whether this duration could be shortened, with a number of trials suggesting that a shorter duration, such as 8 weeks, may be reasonable, but further studies are required to confirm this suggestion [27].

The recent publication of guidelines by the World Health Organization and by the Centers of Disease Control and Prevention (CDC) have assisted in standardising approaches to the prevention of surgical site infections, including prosthetic joint infection [10, 28, 29]. The guidelines have examined the evidence for a number of pre-, intra-, and postoperative strategies to prevent infection and provided graded recommendations. In addition to optimisation of patient comorbidities, preoperative recommended prevention strategies include decolonisation of carriers of *Staphylococcus aureus*, skin antisepsis with alcohol-based skin disinfectants, and administration of surgical antimicrobial prophylaxis within 120 min prior to skin incision, ideally 60 min for short-acting antimicrobials such as cefazolin [29]. Areas in which further evidence is required were also highlighted, including the best approach to managing immunosuppressive therapy preoperatively [29, 30]. Intraoperatively, there was strong support for maintenance of homeostasis, including normothermia, normovolaemia, oxygenation, and glycaemic control [28, 30]. In addition, the use of a single dose of surgical antimicrobial prophylaxis and avoidance of prolonged postoperative antimicrobial prophylaxis was highlighted [28]. The CDC also included specific recommendations for joint replacement surgery [10]. In addition to guidance on the management of immunosuppressive therapy and antimicrobial prophylaxis duration, particularly in the setting of drain tubes, these guidelines examined the evidence for blood transfusion, anticoagulation, orthopaedic space suits, and antimicrobial loaded cements [10].

The importance of research strategies to optimise prevention, diagnosis, and management of prosthetic joint infection continues to be the focus of a significant body of research. As noted in the CDC guidelines, this focus is justified as this is an area of clinical practice 'in which the human and financial burden is greatest' [10]. The landscape in this area of medicine is changing and will continue to do so, particularly in the era of increasingly constrained healthcare budgets and the looming threat of antimicrobial resistance [31, 32]. Concerted, multinational research efforts instill optimism that the early clinical and health economics success of this surgery will continue into the future.

References

1. Gomez PF, Morcuende JA. Early attempts at hip arthroplasty— 1700s to 1950s. Iowa Orthop J. 2005;25:25–9.
2. Kurtz SM, Ong KL, Lau E, Bozic KJ. Impact of the economic downturn on total joint replacement demand in the United States: updated projections to 2021. J Bone Joint Surg Am. 2014;96(8):624–30.
3. Rennert-May E, Bush K, Vickers D, Smith S. Use of a provincial surveillance system to characterize postoperative surgical site infections after primary hip and knee arthroplasty in Alberta, Canada. Am J Infect Control. 2016;44(11):1310–4.
4. Australian Orthopaedic Association. National Joint Replacement Registry. https://aoanjrr.dmac.adelaide.edu.au/. Accessed 3 Oct 2016.
5. Nwachukwu BU, Bozic KJ, Schairer WW, Bernstein JL, Jevsevar DS, Marx RG, Padgett DE. Current status of cost utility analyses in total joint arthroplasty: a systematic review. Clin Orthop Relat Res. 2015;473(5):1815–27.
6. Kent P, McDonald M, Harris O, Mason T, Spelman D. Post-discharge surgical wound infection surveillance in a provincial hospital: Follow-up rates, validity of data and review of the literature. ANZ J Surg. 2001;71(10):583–9.

7. Witso E. The rate of prosthetic joint infection is underestimated in the arthroplasty registers. Acta Orthop. 2015;86(3):277–8.

8. Jamsen E, Huotari K, Huhtala H, Nevalainen J, Konttinen YT. Low rate of infected knee replacements in a nationwide series – is it an underestimate? Acta Orthop. 2009;80(2):205–12.

9. Grammatico-Guillon L, Rusch E, Astagneau P. Surveillance of prosthetic joint infections: international overview and new insights for hospital databases. J Hosp Infect. 2015;89(2):90–8.

10. Berríos-Torres SI, Umscheid CA, Bratzler DW, Leas B, Stone EC, Kelz RR, Healthcare Infection Control Practices Advisory Committee, et al. Centers for Disease Control and Prevention guideline for the prevention of surgical site infection. JAMA Surg. 2017. https://doi.org/10.1001/jamasurg.2017.0904. [Epub ahead of print]

11. Zimmerli W, Trampuz A, Ochsner PE. Prosthetic-joint infections. N Engl J Med. 2004;351(16):1645–54.

12. Benito N, Franco M, Ribera A, Soriano A, Rodriguez-Pardo D, Sorlí L, REIPI (Spanish Network for Research in Infectious Disease) Group for the Study of Prosthetic Joint Infections, et al. Time trends in the aetiology of prosthetic joint infections: a multicentre cohort study. Clin Microbiol Infect. 2016;22:732.e1–8.

13. Parvizi J, Gehrke T, Musculoskeletal Infection Society. Proceedings of the International Consensus on Periprosthetic Joint Infection. 2013. http://www.msis-na.org/wp-content/themes/msis-temp/pdf/ism-periprosthetic-joint-information.pdf. Accessed 7 Feb 2017.

14. Tsukayama DT, Estrada R, Gustilo RB. Infection after total hip arthroplasty. A study of the treatment of one hundred and six infections. J Bone Joint Surg. 1996;78(4):512–23.

15. Barrett L, Atkins B. The clinical presentation of prosthetic joint infection. J Antimicrob Chemother. 2014;69(Suppl 1):i25–7.

16. Atkins B, Athanasou N, Deeks J, Crook D, Simpson H, Peto T, The OSIRIS Collaborative Study Group, et al. Prospective evaluation of criteria for microbiological diagnosis of prosthetic-joint infection at revision arthroplasty. J Clin Microbiol. 1998;36(10):2932–9.

17. Osmon D, Berbari E, Berendt A, Lew D, Zimmerli W, Steckelberg J, Infectious Diseases Society of America, et al. Diagnosis and management of prosthetic joint infection: clinical practice guidelines by the Infectious Diseases Society of America. Clin Infect Dis. 2013;56(1):e1–e25.

18. Parvizi J, Gehrke T, International Consensus Group on Periprosthetic Joint Infection. Definition of periprosthetic joint infection. J Arthroplasty. 2014;29(7):1331.

19. Aggarwal VK, Higuera C, Deirmengian G, Parvizi J, Austin MS. Swab cultures are not as effective as tissue cultures for diagnosis of periprosthetic joint infection. Clin Orthop Relat Res. 2013;471(10):3196–203.

20. Trampuz A, Piper KE, Jacobson MJ, Hanssen AD, Unni KK, Osmon DR, et al. Sonication of removed hip and knee prostheses for diagnosis of infection. N Engl J Med. 2007;357(7):654–63.

21. Peel TN, Dylla BL, Hughes JG, Lynch DT, Greenwood-Quaintance KE, Cheng AC, et al. Improved diagnosis of prosthetic joint infection by culturing periprosthetic tissue specimens in blood culture bottles. MBio. 2016;7(1):e01776–15.

22. Hughes HC, Newnham R, Athanasou N, Atkins BL, Bejon P, Bowler IC. Microbiological diagnosis of prosthetic joint infections: a prospective evaluation of four bacterial culture media in the routine laboratory. Clin Microbiol Infect. 2011;17(10):1528–30.

23. Hughes JG, Vetter EA, Patel R, Schleck CD, Harmsen S, Turgeant LT, Cockerill FR 3rd. Culture with BACTEC Peds Plus/F bottle compared with conventional methods for detection of bacteria in synovial fluid. J Clin Microbiol. 2001;39(12):4468–71.

24. Peel TN, Spelman T, Dylla BL, Hughes JG, Greenwood-Quaintance KE, Cheng AC, et al. Optimal periprosthetic tissue specimen number for diagnosis of prosthetic joint infection. J Clin Microbiol. 2017;55(1):234–43.

25. Bémer P, Leger J, Tande D, Plouzeau C, Valentin AS, Jolivet-Gougeon A, et al. How many samples and how many culture media to diagnose a prosthetic joint infection: a clinical and microbiological prospective multicenter study. J Clin Microbiol. 2016;54(2):385–91.

26. Deirmengian C, Kardos K, Kilmartin P, Cameron A, Schiller K, Parvizi J. Diagnosing periprosthetic joint infection: has the era of the biomarker arrived? Clin Orthop Relat Res. 2014;472(11):3254–62.

27. Lora-Tamayo J, Euba G, Cobo J, Horcajada JP, Soriano A, Sandoval E, Prosthetic Joint Infection Group of the Spanish Network for Research in Infectious Diseases—REIPI, et al. Short- versus long-duration levofloxacin plus rifampicin for acute staphylococcal prosthetic joint infection managed with implant retention: a randomised clinical trial. Int J Antimicrob Agents. 2016;48(3):310–6.

28. Allegranzi B, Zayed B, Bischoff P, Kubilay NZ, de Jonge S, de Vries F, WHO Guidelines Development Group, et al. New WHO recommendations on intraoperative and postoperative measures for surgical site infection prevention: an evidence-based global perspective. Lancet Infect Dis. 2016;16(12):e288–303.
29. Allegranzi B, Bischoff P, de Jonge S, Kubilay NZ, Zayed B, Gomes SM, WHO Guidelines Development Group, et al. New WHO recommendations on preoperative measures for surgical site infection prevention: an evidence-based global perspective. Lancet Infect Dis. 2016;16:e276–87.
30. Berrios-Torres SI, Yi SH, Bratzler DW, Ma A, Mu Y, Zhu L, Jernigan JA. Activity of commonly used antimicrobial prophylaxis regimens against pathogens causing coronary artery bypass graft and arthroplasty surgical site infections in the United States, 2006-2009. Infect Control Hosp Epidemiol. 2014;35(3):231–9.
31. Fournier PE, Drancourt M, Colson P, Rolain JM, La Scola B, Raoult D. Modern clinical microbiology: new challenges and solutions. Nat Rev Microbiol. 2013;11(8):574–85.
32. Review on Antimicrobial Resistance. Antimicrobial resistance: tackling a crisis for the health and wealth of nations. 2014; London: UK Government and Wellcome Trust. https://amr-review.org/home.html. Accessed 30 Jun 2017.

Index

© Springer International Publishing AG 2018   257
T. Peel (ed.), *Prosthetic Joint Infections*,
https://doi.org/10.1007/978-3-319-65250-4